The Recipes of
Champions

Nutritional Secrets
of 100 Canadian Olympians

By Martin Glynn et al

Macmillan Canada
Toronto

Dedication

For Peggy Glynn, my mother, who always told me I could do anything.

For Martin Glynn, my father, who always told me to do it right.

For my son Matt who is a constant reminder of all that is good in the world. Bless you.

For my brothers and sisters who are always there.

Canadian Cataloguing in Publication Data

Main entry under title:

The recipes of champions: Nutritional secrets of 100 Canadian Olympians

Includes index.
ISBN 0-7715-7630-7

1. Cookery. I. Glynn, Martin.

TX714.R434 1998   641.5   C98-931856-7

This book is available at special discounts for bulk purchases by your group or organization for sales promotions, premiums, fundraising and seminars. For details, contact: Macmillan Canada, Special Sales Department, 29 Birch Avenue, Toronto, ON M4V 1E2. Tel: 416-963-8830.

Martin Glynn Associates Inc.
130 Lauder Avenue
Toronto ON Canada M6H 3E5
E-Mail: swim@ican.net

Printed in Canada by Transcontinental Printing Inc.

The Recipes of Champions

contents

In support of

unicef

Acknowledgments

To the athletes and agents who said, "yes"; to all those who have crossed my path on this journey; to all those who have said "Great initiative!"; to all those who have said "Good job!"; to all those who have lent support to the project; to those who have been keenly involved; and to those who have known me intimately during this two year odyssey...the job is done, and I love you all.

Martin Glynn

August 15, 1998

Suschitra Powell

Omar Brooks

Greg Muir

Donna Muir

Carrie Roy

Martha Buchanan

Sylvia Doucette

Lisa Diamond

Irene Schachtler

Tom Boreskie

Richard Stamper

Tom Scanlon

Mike Hines

Peter Maher

Sandy Grant

Jim Meikle and the Brampton Print Group

Dr. K. G. Koski

Brian Cooper

Jim Boyle

Jean Lambert

Brian Gilligan

Joanne Gray

Laurent Larose

Marie Maltais

Theresa Allum

Ron Besse and the Macmillan family

Christine McDowell

Yves Paquette and all the team at The Canadian Sporting Goods Association

Dick Pound

Peter Schleicher and everyone at Swiss Air

Bonnie Stern

Rick Turnbull

Andrea Thibault

Bill Hushion and the folks at Hushion House

Dave Best

Laurie Swim

Paul Herbert

Ron Lieberman

Linda Curatolo

Michael Chow

EDITORIAL

John McCormick

Mary Patton

Brenda Whiteway

Larry Goldstein

FOOD PREPARATION & RECIPE TESTING

David Wolfman

Jen Sladek

Chris Lane

Eshun Mott

Christine Crawszyk

PHOTOGRAPHY

All food photography Pete Herlihy, Orangeville, Ontario.

All athletes' photos courtesy of Canadian Sport Images, Ottawa, Ontario, except where otherwise noted.

PRODUCTION & DESIGN

John Kerr

Jim Stubbington

Angie Brega

Dejan Kocetkov

Jennifer Swatten

Josie Lomon

Bob & Karen Paul of Weathervane Studios

"Life is no brief candle for me. It is a sort of splendid torch which I have got hold of for the moment, and I want to make it burn as brightly as possible before handing it on to future generations."

– George Bernard Shaw

An Ancient Tradition Reborn

Some 2700 years ago, all wars ceased during the Greek Olympiads as part of the custom of *ekecheiria*, the Olympic Truce, so that athletes and spectators could travel safely to and from the competitions. In the late 19th century, French aristocrat Pierre de Coubertin gave birth to the vision of 'world harmony through sports', and international sport competition once again became a vehicle for the peaceful coming together of all nations and peoples. Today, along with the fanfare, the corporate logos and the dreams of glory, the Games continue to be a venue where the world community unites in the pursuit of excellence and peaceful competition.

Ekecheiria inspired a 1992 United Nations resolution to ban war during the Olympic Games. This would allow UNICEF field workers the opportunity to take advantage of the lull in the fighting to bring much-needed assistance to children in war-torn countries. In a similar spirit, Olympic athletes themselves understand that the modern version of the Olympics is about far more than winning medals. Many are volunteers who help generate financial assistance for those in need, especially in Olympic years.

Tying together the themes of peace and service was Atlanta Olympic Aid, a program created to increase awareness and raise money to help UNICEF in its relief efforts. As an Olympian and a long-time volunteer for the Canadian Olympic Association (COA), I was asked to lead the initiative in Canada. Thus, during the 1996 Games in Atlanta, I began approaching fellow Olympians for support. With their help and the generous advice of many experts, *The Recipes of Champions* came into being.

A portion of the proceeds from the sale of this book will go to UNICEF for its work in advancing children's rights to survival, protection and development in peace and in war, and to the COA for its work in support of athletes' programs.

Martin Glynn, August 1998

Foreword

by Olympic Coach Andy Higgins

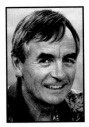

Recipes are directions that give variety to the nourishing of our bodies, sustaining life. A portion of the proceeds from this book will go to UNICEF, whose purpose is to nourish the hearts, minds and bodies of the world's most vulnerable children.

This book is also a reminder that each one of us can make a difference.

Every time we use this book, we shall remember that we each have much to be thankful for, that every small act of kindness and generosity can make an immense difference, and that when we approach food with this awareness it nourishes our heart and soul as well as our bodies.

The Recipes of Champions exemplifies what I believe to be the Olympian attitude, and it can be expressed by every single one of us, for each of us is gifted, although in different ways.

A few of us have been given a world class gift: The caring heart of an Albert Schweitzer, the compassionate soul of a Mother Theresa, the music that was Mozart, the nervous system and muscles of Donovan Bailey. Those who become Olympians have been given a special gift by their Creator and they are able to express that gift at the highest levels of competition because they consciously choose an attitude that supports their positive growth.

Every single one of us, however, because we are human, has been given one equal, and magnificent gift. It is the gift of a dream. What we do with that gift is choose. Victor Frankl, Holocaust survivor and author of *Man's Search for Meaning*, wrote, "man's ultimate freedom is to choose his attitude."

Martin Glynn, an Olympian and the driving force of this book, has made that choice and lives it continuously. He created a way for Olympians to help UNICEF in its work of saving and improving children's lives.

Learning to "give away" is a particularly human challenge. It is central to the spiritual teachings of the First Nations, and it is at the heart of all spiritual systems. It is no surprise then that Olympians, who themselves struggle to overcome their own limitations of attitude and belief, have a strong sense of needing to give something back to their community.

Inherent in the attitude of Olympians is an awareness that while they were alone in the competitive arena, they did not get there by themselves. Thus the sense of wanting to give something back.

This book is the result of small generous actions by many people. It is a demonstration of the truth that all of us is stronger than any of us.

Inspiration is the real value of Olympians to the community. Every heart and soul is touched by human excellence expressed in both body and spirit. At a deep level our being is inspired to ask that ultimately moving human question: "am I reaching for my ultimate potential?" This is the question that unsettles our complacency, causes us to question and to begin anew the change and growth process.

Everyone, including Martin, the Olympic amateur chefs, the many volunteers who gave so freely of their expertise, and all who purchase *The Recipes of Champions*, are making a difference. You are helping to save and to improve innocent lives, by supporting UNICEF. It is my hope that this book, for all who use it, will become a tangible reminder of our option to choose an Olympian attitude and to express it in every aspect of our lives.

For 35 years Andy Higgins was a hugely popular teacher and highly successful coach, supporting athletes to the podium in every major game for which Canadians were eligible, including David Steen, Olympics '88, and Michael Smith, World Championships '91. Since 1995 Andy has been a speaker and coach in the corporate world. He may be reached by email at: coachajhig@aol.com

Nutritious Choices for High Energy

by Elizabeth Mansfield

Olympic athletes know which foods and beverages are crucial to optimal health and peak performance. For those who are less certain, some general rules of thumb apply. To perform at your peak you need to pay attention to what you eat and drink. Canada's Food Guide, developed by and available from Health Canada gives you an Action Plan for Daily Food Choices. It's important to eat a wide variety of foods from each of the food groups because each food group has specific essential nutrients that you need for your good health and athletic performance.

Whole grains, breads and cereals are rich in carbohydrates, B vitamins, iron and fibre; fruits and vegetables are chock full of vitamins and minerals, fibre and carbohydrate; milk products are key sources of calcium, riboflavin, vitamin D and protein; and meats and alternatives are our major sources of protein, iron, zinc, and vitamin B_{12}. In moderation, all foods fit into a sport nutrition action plan, but throughout your day choose foods that are rich in carbohydrates because these are your best energy foods.

Examples of carbohydrate rich food selections from within each Food Group:

Breads & Cereals	Fruits & Vegetables	Milk & Milk Products	Meats & Alternatives
cereals	raisins, apricots	fruit yogurts	chilli with kidney beans
breads	fruit juices, fruit smoothies	chocolate milk, milk based puddings	French Canadian pea soup
rice, pasta	potatoes, beets, carrots, corn	lower fat ice cream or frozen yogurt	lentil casserole

Guidelines for Healthy Eating

- Enjoy a variety of foods
- Emphasise cereals, breads, other grain products, vegetables and fruits
- Choose lower fat dairy products, leaner meats and foods prepared with little or no fat
- Limit salt, alcohol, and caffeine

Take Action with your Sport Nutrition

Before practice or competition:

Be well hydrated and fuelled before your training and competitions so that you can perform at your best.

Drink at least 10-12 cups of fluid a day to meet your body's daily fluid needs.

Drink at least two cups (500 mL) of fluid within the two hours before training or competition.

To be sure you are drinking enough fluid check your urine. Lots of clear, almost colourless urine means that you are ready to play.

- Choose high-octane fuel in the form of complex carbohydrates to keep you tanked up and ready to perform. Choose cereals and breads for breakfast. Order sandwiches on whole grain breads such as whole wheat, multigrain, pumpernickel or rye for lunch. Be adventurous; try different grains for supper once in a while, like couscous, bulghur or brown rice. Use beans and peas such as chick peas, lentils, or kidney beans in salads, soups and casseroles.

• Score bonus points with fruits and vegetables. For a wide variety of nutrients choose the brightly coloured fruits and vegetables more often. Start off your day with a glass of juice in the morning or a small piece of fruit. Start at least one meal a day with a salad or cut up vegies.

• Make it a habit to drink at least one cup of 1% or skim milk every day.

• Choose one dairy snack such as cheese or yogurt each day and try to have cereal with milk 3-5 times a week at breakfast.

• Meat products are a great source of iron, which helps carry oxygen to the working muscles. Choose lean cuts of meat and poultry such as round steaks, lean ground beef, veal, pork, and skinless chicken breast. Choose fish that has been broiled, grilled, steamed, baked or poached rather than fried.

During practice or competition:

Don't wait until you are thirsty to drink; you may already be dehydrated. Bring your own water bottle and keep it topped up. Drink every 15 minutes even if you are not thirsty. When you're thirsty, drink until you are not thirsty and then drink a little more. Try to drink as much as you can tolerate during your activity. Though water is best, a sports drink can be a good choice too as it supplies energy and electrolytes that encourage you to drink by "turning on" your thirst. This helps you to drink more and stay well hydrated and fuelled during your practice or game. Watch for these signs of dehydration:

Warning Signs of Dehydration:
   • dizziness and light-headedness, poor concentration • muscle cramps • nausea and headache

Chronic Signs of Dehydration:
   • loss of appetite • dark yellow urine, little or even no urine • muscle cramps

After practice or competition:

This is one of the most important times to refuel and rehydrate. To make sure that you drink enough fluid, drink two cups (500 mL) for each pound (0.5kg) of weight that you lose during training or competition.

Help your muscles to recover even faster and stock up on all that used-up muscle energy by eating and/or drinking within 15-30 minutes after training or competition. Choose carbohydrate rich beverages such as fruit juices or fruit drinks, sport drinks, or soda pop; and/or carbohydrate rich foods such as bagels and jam, low fat fruit yogurts, and fresh or canned fruits. You should also eat a high carbohydrate meal by the end of each training day to promote adequate recovery.

REMEMBER...YOU'LL ONLY GO AS FAR AS YOUR NUTRITION WILL TAKE YOU!

Elizabeth (Beth) Mansfield, MSc, RD is a nutrition and exercise specialist with EDM Peak Performance in Ottawa. She develops training and nutrition programs for professional, elite and recreational athletes in Canada and the USA. For more nutrition and exercise information check out the EDM Peak Performance website at http://infoweb.magi.com/~edm/

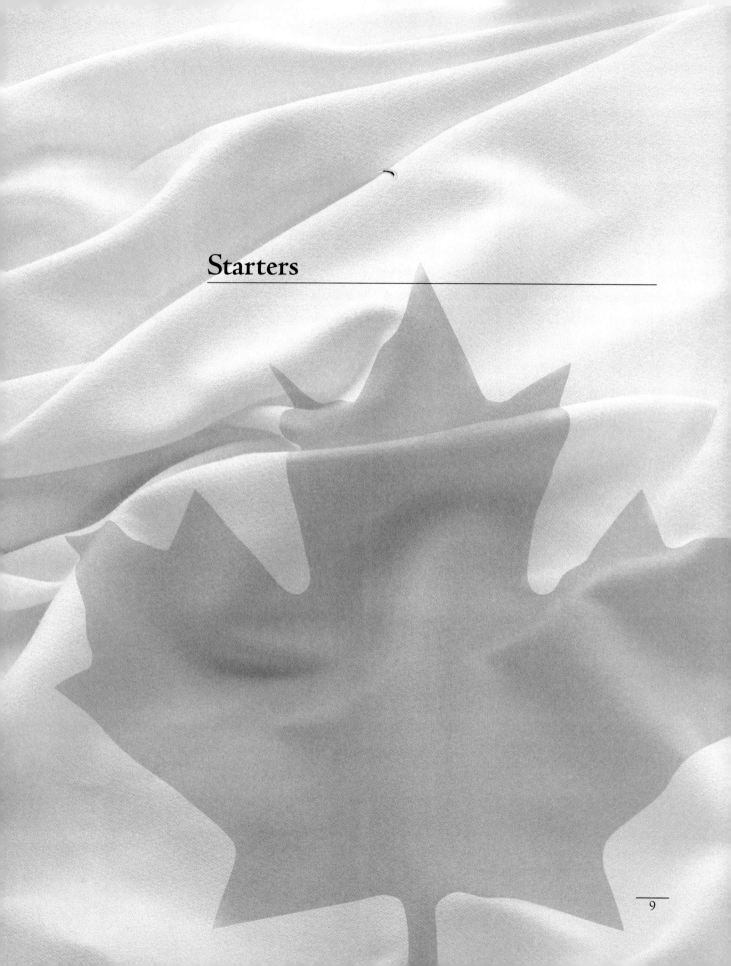

Starters

9

Sheryl's Monster Muesli

Preparation time: 15 minutes

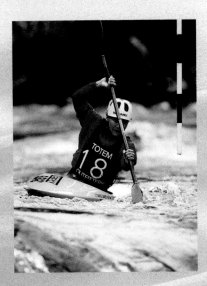

Sheryl Boyle
C A N O E I N G

Building on her victories in slalom canoeing at the Canadian championships in 1993, 1994 and 1996, Sheryl went to the 1996 Olympics with high expectations. She did not disappoint, winning a silver medal in Atlanta, and has emerged as the best female slalom paddler in Canada and is among the top-ranked in the world. Sheryl, whose hometown is Bonnechere, Ontario, is pursuing a master's degree in architectural history and theory at McGill University.

Sheryl says, "This is my favourite peak-performance breakfast because it helps me get a good start to the day. And boy, is it real fibre or what! It's also high in protein and carbohydrates and low in fat."

5 cups	large-flake rolled oats	1.25 L
1½ cups	spelt flakes	375 mL
¾ cup	rye flakes	150 mL
½ cup	wheat flakes	125 mL
½ cup	barley flakes	125 mL
1 cup	chopped hazelnuts	250 mL
1 cup	thinly shaved almonds	250 mL
½ cup	dried cranberries	125 mL
1 cup	unsalted sunflower seeds	250 mL
1½ cups	raisins	375 mL
1 Tbsp.	amaranth seeds	15 mL

In a large bowl, combine all ingredients except raisins and amaranth seeds. Put the raisins in a large plastic container with a lid, and add a few drops of water to make them sticky. Pour amaranth seeds onto raisins, close container and shake; seeds will stick to raisins. Add raisin mixture to muesli, and mix well. Serve ½ cup (125 ml) muesli with ½ cup (125 ml) hot low-fat milk or yogurt. Serves 25.

Nutritional values per serving
(based on 25 servings):
calories: 177
fat: 10 g; 51% of calories
protein: 6 g; 13% of calories
carbohydrates: 16 g; 37% of calories

Sheryl's Performance Eating Tip:

The key to being lean and strong is a low-fat, high-fibre diet.

More Than Muesli

Preparation time: 15 minutes

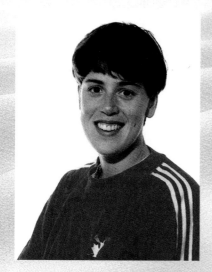

Anna Van Der Kamp
R O W I N G

Anna grew up in Vancouver and Port Hardy, British Columbia. She played virtually every sport that was available to her, but in her second year at the University of Victoria, when she joined the novice rowing team, she knew she'd found her sport. Anna rowed for the university for four years and first made the national team in 1994. In Atlanta, they won silver in the women's 8+.

After years of going to Europe to race and train and enjoying the muesli, Anna decided to take the idea home with her. It fits in well with her diet, is easily digested and covers several nutritional basics. In race season, this is a good morning meal—a small serving a few hours before a race will satisfy hunger. During training, it is a terrific snack between or after workouts. You can substitute different fruits (kiwi, banana, mango, etc.) and sweeteners (instead of sugar, try honey, flavoured yogurt or sweetened granola).

2 cups	plain yogurt	500 mL
I	apple, quartered	I
I	pear, quartered	I
¼ cup	brown sugar	50 mL
¾ cup	oatmeal	150 mL
½ cup	raisins	125 mL
I cup	granola	250 mL
I tsp.	coconut	5 mL
¼ tsp.	cinnamon	I mL

Put yogurt into a container that will hold at least 4 cups (I L). Grate the apple and pear into the yogurt. Add remaining ingredients, and stir. Keep refrigerated. The muesli tends to go brown and mushy after a day or so, but that doesn't affect the taste. It will keep for several days in the refrigerator. Serves 4.

Nutritional values per serving
(based on 4 servings):

calories: 436

fat: 13 g; 28% of calories

protein: 11 g; 10% of calories

carbohydrates: 68 g; 62% of calories

Oatmeal Made Palatable

Preparation time: 10 minutes

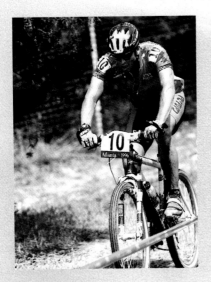

Andreas likes this version of oatmeal because it is an excellent energy source, high in carbohydrates. He usually eats it before an event. Dried pineapple or mango can be substituted for raisins. Rice Dream is a rice beverage available in natural-food stores.

⅓ cup	quick-cooking oatmeal, preferably organic	75 mL
¾ cup	boiling water	150 mL
1 Tbsp.	sunflower seeds	15 mL
1 Tbsp.	raisins	15 mL
1 tsp.	flaxseed oil	5 mL

Add oatmeal to boiling water, and cook for about 5 minutes. Cool slightly, and add remaining ingredients. Serve with Rice Dream instead of milk, and top with maple syrup or molasses. Serves 1.

Andreas Hestler
C Y C L I N G

Andreas has been cycling for eight years and is a two-time Canada Cup winner (1994 and 1995). In 1995, he was the national champion and, in 1996, won the Cactus Cup and was on the Olympic team. He enjoys healthy eating and believes in the "organic way."

Nutritional values per serving
(based on 1 serving; without Rice Dream, maple syrup or molasses):

calories: 234

fat: 11 g; 43% of calories

protein: 6 g; 11% of calories

carbohydrates: 27 g; 46% of calories

Andreas' Performance Eating Tip:

Dairy products in combination with grains change the rate of absorption. Typically, oatmeal with milk results in a "heavy stomach," a problem you can avoid by using Rice Dream instead.

Rower's Delight

Preparation time: 15 minutes

Maria says this is her favourite dish because it tastes terrific, is easy to prepare and is definitely a crowd pleaser. She usually eats it after her first workout of the morning (one of three per day). This meal will keep you going all day.

I loaf	fresh unsliced white bread	I loaf
3	eggs	3
I cup	skim milk	250 mL

Cut the bread into thick slices. Beat eggs in a shallow bowl, and stir in milk. Dip bread in egg-milk mixture, turning each piece to make sure the liquid soaks in on both sides. Cook in preheated frying pan over medium heat until lightly browned on both sides. Serve with desired toppings (brown sugar, cinnamon, syrup, fresh fruit or anything else you like). Serves 6.

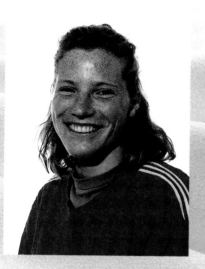

Maria Maunder
R O W I N G

Maria won silver medals in the women's 8+ at the 1996 Olympic Games and in the Rotsee Regatta in Lucerne, Switzerland. She is currently in the M.B.A. program at Concordia University in Montreal. Her other interests include reading, skiing and swimming.

Nutritional values per serving
(based on 6 servings):
calories: 63
fat: 3 g; 39% of calories
protein: 5 g; 31% of calories
carbohydrates: 5 g; 30% of calories

Maria's Performance Eating Tip:

Eating well is the key to top performance.

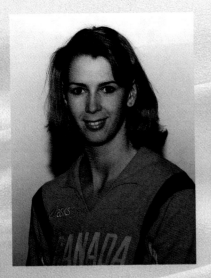

Kathy Tough
V O L L E Y B A L L

In 1996, Kathy was named captain of the Canadian Women's Olympic Volleyball Team and her team made history when it became the first Canadian women's volleyball team to win a match at the Olympics. This was a highlight in Kathy's 13-year career in volleyball. Atlanta also marked the end of Kathy's indoor career, but she shows no signs of relaxing. She's heading for the beach, where she plans to play beach volleyball and compete at the international level.

Kathy is an exercise therapist at the Canadian Back Institute. She has a B.P.E. from the University of Calgary and is a public speaker for drug-free sport.

Nutritional values per pancake
(based on 18 pancakes):
calories: 94
fat: 2 g; 24% of calories
protein: 3 g; 13% of calories
carbohydrates: 15 g; 63% of calories

Perfect Pancakes

Preparation time: 15 minutes

Pancakes that are "tough" to beat—here's the family's secret recipe.

2 cups	flour	500 mL
4 tsp.	baking powder	20 mL
pinch	salt	pinch
4 Tbsp.	sugar	50 mL
2 cups	2% milk	500 mL
2	eggs	2
2 Tbsp.	butter or margarine	25 mL

Combine flour, baking powder, salt and sugar, and mix well. In a separate bowl, mix together milk and eggs. Add dry ingredients to liquid ingredients, and stir until blended. Add butter or margarine last. Drop onto heated, oiled frying pan. Cook over medium heat on one side until the batter stops bubbling on top, then flip and cook the other side. Makes about 18 4-inch (10 cm) pancakes.

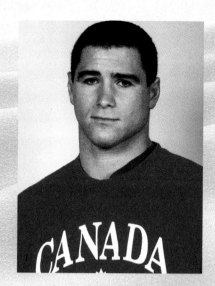

Colbie Bell
W R E S T L I N G

In 1996, Colbie placed 1st in the 100-kg class at the Canadian nationals in Greco-Roman wrestling, 3rd in the Canadian nationals in freestyle and 4th in the Pan American Games in Greco-Roman. An animal sciences student at the University of Alberta, he also enjoys sailing and scuba diving.

Healthy Pancakes

Preparation time: 15 minutes

Colbie says these pancakes are among his favourites because they are low in fat (important for weigh-ins) and taste good, especially for breakfast.

4	egg whites	4
2 Tbsp.	pancake mix	25 mL
¾ cup	uncooked oatmeal	150 mL
2 Tbsp.	raisins	25 mL
¼ tsp.	vanilla	1 mL
¼ cup	strawberries	50 mL
1 tsp.	cinnamon	5 mL

Combine all ingredients in a blender. Pour mixture into a nonstick frying pan at medium heat. Cook until batter stops bubbling, then flip and cook the other side. Makes 8 4-inch (10 cm) pancakes.

Nutritional values per pancake
(based on 8 pancakes):
calories: 52
fat: 0.5 g; 8% of calories
protein: 3 g; 24% of calories
carbohydrates: 9 g; 67% of calories

Sandra Schmirler's Power Pancakes

Preparation time: 10 minutes

"My husband, Shannon, is really the cook in the family, and he modified this basic pancake recipe to use healthier ingredients."

3	egg whites	3
1¾ cups	skim milk	400 mL
1 Tbsp.	olive oil	15 mL
1 cup	all-purpose flour	250 mL
¾ cup	whole wheat	150 mL
2 containers	fat-free yogurt, any flavour	350 g
4 tsp.	baking powder	20 mL
½ tsp.	salt	2 mL

Mix all ingredients together. Fry in a non-stick frying pan so that you don't need much oil. Serves 12.

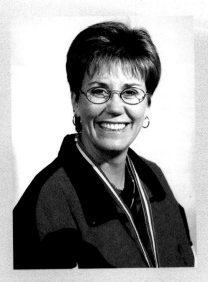

Sandra Schmirler
C U R L I N G

"I guess we're consistent, and we play hard, and we never give up...that makes a difference," says Sandra. Being the Skip for the best team in women's curling history, she knows whereof she speaks. Before going to Nagano, Sandra and her team competed in six provincial championships, three national championships, and three world championships. She is currently a supervisor at the South East Leisure Centre in Regina. Born 34 years ago in Biggar, Saskatchewan, she has been curling for 22 years.

Nutritional values per serving
(based on 12 servings):
calories: 83
fat: 2 g; 24% of calories
protein: 4 g; 20% of calories
carbohydrates: 11 g; 55% of calories

Sandra's Training Tip:

Don't just set a goal, set a dream. We all know that dreams do come true, and it is far more enchanting to live out a dream!

All-Canadian Bannock

Preparation time: 45 minutes

Cari says this is her favourite peak-performance food because it is easy to prepare, very tasty, a great vehicle for honey and low in fat. She normally eats bannock after a five-hour practice. Raisins, blueberries or cranberries can be added to the dough.

3 cups	all-purpose flour	750 mL
1 tsp.	salt	5 mL
2 Tbsp.	baking powder	25 mL
¼ cup	margarine, melted	50 mL
1½ cups	water	375 mL

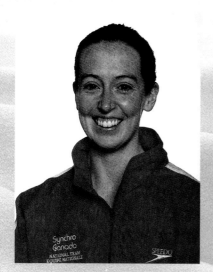

Cari Read
SYNCHRONIZED SWIMMING

Cari is a nine-year member of the Canadian national team. She won silver at the 1996 Atlanta Olympics in the synchronized swimming team event and, in 1993, was the Canadian duet champion.

Combine flour, salt and baking powder in a large bowl. In a separate bowl, pour melted margarine into water, then add to dry ingredients. Mix with fork, form into a ball, and knead gently 10 times on a floured surface. Pat into a ½-inch-thick (2 cm) circle. Cook in lightly oiled frying pan over medium heat for 15 minutes on each side. Don't try to cook it faster — if the heat is above medium, the bannock will burn on the outside and remain uncooked inside. Use two lifters for turning. Serve hot. Serves 10.

Nutritional values per serving
(based on 10 servings):
calories: 177
fat: 5 g; 25% of calories
protein: 4 g; 9% of calories
carbohydrates: 29 g; 66% of calories

Cari's Performance Eating Tip:

Eat all four food groups, especially whole grains and fruits.

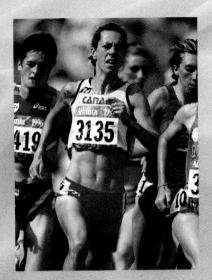

Leah Pells
R U N N I N G

The Canadian mile record holder at 4:23, Leah is ranked number one in Canada and North America in both the 1,500-metre and the mile and among the top five in the world in the 1,500-metre. She wants to be the best middle-distance runner Canada has ever produced.

Leah continues to pursue excellence in her sport and has her sights set on the 2000 Olympics in Sydney, Australia. She is a part-time child-care counsellor and a member of The Esteem Team, a group of athletes who talk to schoolchildren about peer pressure and making positive choices.

Grandma's Scones

Preparation time: 30 minutes

Leah says these scones are her favourite food because they taste wonderful and are light and easy to digest. They're good with homemade strawberry jam and especially tasty fresh out of the oven. She eats them three hours before a race.

2 cups	flour	500 mL
½ cup	shortening	125 mL
½ cup	sugar	125 mL
½ tsp.	salt	2 mL
1 cup	currants	250 mL
1	egg, beaten	1
2½ tsp.	baking powder	12 mL
¼ tsp.	baking soda	1 mL
1 cup	buttermilk	250 mL

Mix together flour, shortening, sugar and salt. Add remaining ingredients, and mix until dough begins to cling together. Knead gently on lightly floured surface. Pat dough to ½-inch (1 cm) thickness, and cut into desired shape. Place on ungreased cookie sheet, and bake for 15 minutes at 425°F (220°C). Makes about 12 scones.

Leah's Performance Eating Tip:

Eat lots of small meals throughout the day, especially fruits, vegetables and other low-fat foods.

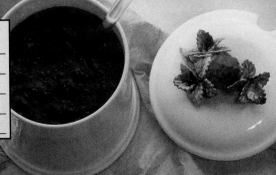

Nutritional values per scone
(based on 12 scones):
calories: 214
fat: 10 g; 43% of calories
protein: 3 g; 6% of calories
carbohydrates: 27 g; 50% of calories

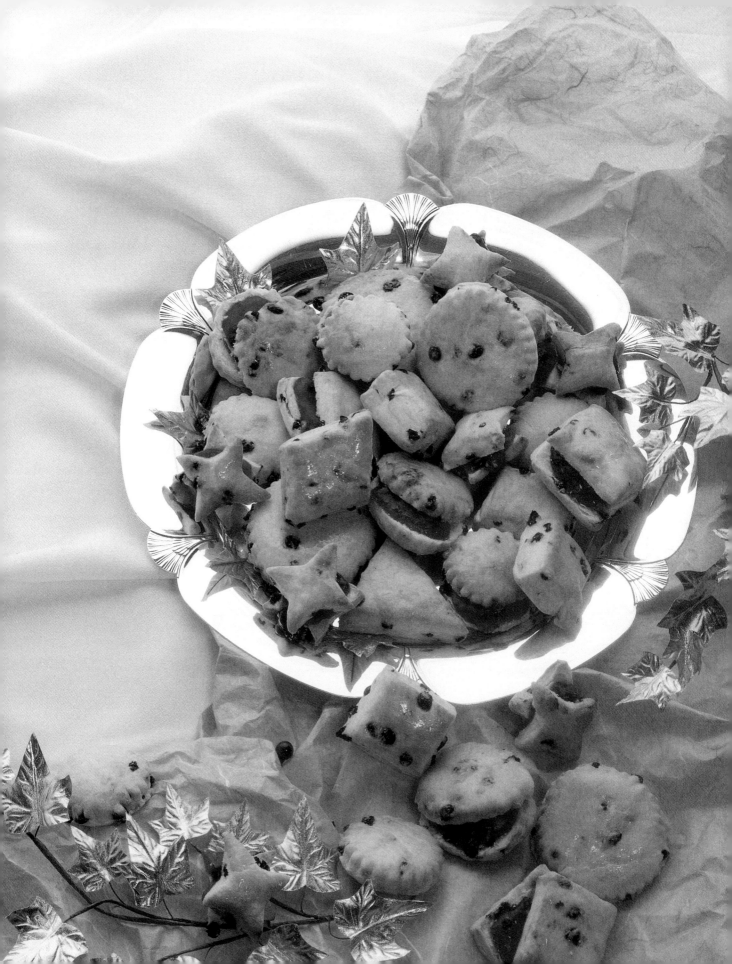

Low-Fat Rhubarb Oatmeal Muffins

Preparation time: 45 minutes

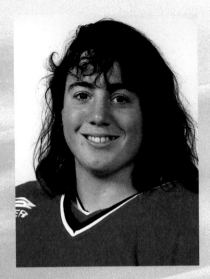

Rebecca Fahey
WOMEN'S
HOCKEY

Originally from Sackville, NB, Rebecca attends the Olympic Oval High Performance Female Hockey Program. From the age of 16, she has competed provincially and nationally, and was a member of the gold-medal-winning Team Canada at the 1995 and 1996 Pacific Rim. She has been involved in Women's varsity soccer at Mount Allison University, and enjoys golfing in her spare time. Her motto: 'No pain, no gain'.

Rebecca loves these muffins for breakfast. They are quick and easy to prepare, and full of good things to start her day.

2 cups	rhubarb pieces (fresh or frozen)	500 mL
2	egg whites	2
1 cup	skim milk	250 mL
1 tsp.	lemon juice	5 mL
½ cup	applesauce or low-fat plain yogurt	125 mL
2½ cups	whole wheat flour	625 mL
2 cups	brown sugar	500 mL
1 cup	rolled oats	250 mL
1 tsp.	cinnamon	5 mL
1 tsp.	baking soda	5 mL
½ tsp.	salt	2 mL

Preheat oven to 350°F (180°C). In a mixing bowl, beat egg whites. Stir in milk, lemon juice and applesauce or yogurt. In another mixing bowl, combine flour, sugar, oats, cinnamon, baking soda, and salt. Blend wet and dry ingredients. Stir in rhubarb. Bake 30-35 minutes.

Nutritional values per serving
(based on 12 servings):
calories: 219
fat: 1 g; 4% of calories
protein: 6 g; 11% of calories
carbohydrates: 47 g; 85% of calories

Morning Riser

Preparation time: 10 minutes

Sandra says this is her favourite peak-performance food because it is quick and easy and a good source of vitamins and minerals. It tastes great and can go anywhere with her. She normally has this drink in the morning before a workout. It's light enough to train on and packs enough calories to keep her going.

I cup	fresh or frozen fruit (anything except kiwi)	250 mL
3 scoops	frozen nonfat yogurt, plain or vanilla	3 scoops
¾ cup	fruit juice of choice	150 mL
½ tsp.	vanilla	2 mL
I	egg (optional)	I

Peel and cut one or two kinds of fruit into cubes or slices, and drop into a blender. Add remaining ingredients, blend until smooth, and pour into a glass. Serves I.

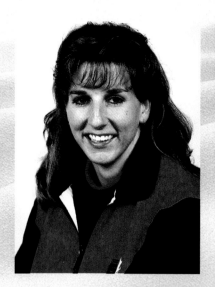

Sandra Beasley
S O F T B A L L

Sandra has been a member of the national team since 1987. She has competed in two world championships (1990 and 1994), two Pan American Games (1991 and 1995) and the 1996 Olympics in Atlanta. She plays left field.

Sandra was born in Delta, British Columbia, and attended Stephen F. Austin State University in Texas on a full scholarship, where she completed a B.Sc. degree. She now lives in Arlington, Texas, where she teaches elementary school.

Nutritional values per serving
(based on 1 serving; includes egg):
calories: 271
fat: 6 g; 21% of calories
protein: 8 g; 13% of calories
carbohydrates: 45 g; 67% of calories

Sandy's Performance Eating Tip:

Make sure your eating habits cover your health needs, not just your schedule.

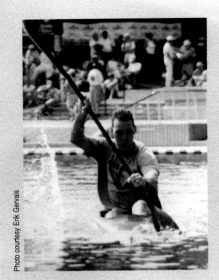

Photo courtesy Erik Gervais

Blender Fruit Drink

Preparation time: 5 minutes

This is a good source of carbohydrates and vitamin C. Erik usually drinks it after a hard practice to replenish fluids.

2-3 cups	apple juice	500-750 mL
I	frozen banana, sliced	I
6-8	frozen strawberries	6-8

Place all ingredients in a blender, and blend until well mixed. Serves 2.

Erik Gervais
C A N O E I N G

Erik, who has been kayaking since he was 11, has won many provincial, national and international awards—50 gold, 15 silver and 10 bronze medals. He participated in the 1995 Pan American Games and the 1996 Olympics in Atlanta. Erik lives in Valleyfield, Quebec, and is currently a student. He plans to specialize in computer-aided design when he completes his studies. His other interests include basketball, hockey, reading and music.

Nutritional values per serving
(based on 2 servings):

calories: 223

fat: I g; 3% of calories

protein: I g; 2% of calories

carbohydrates: 53 g; 95% of calories

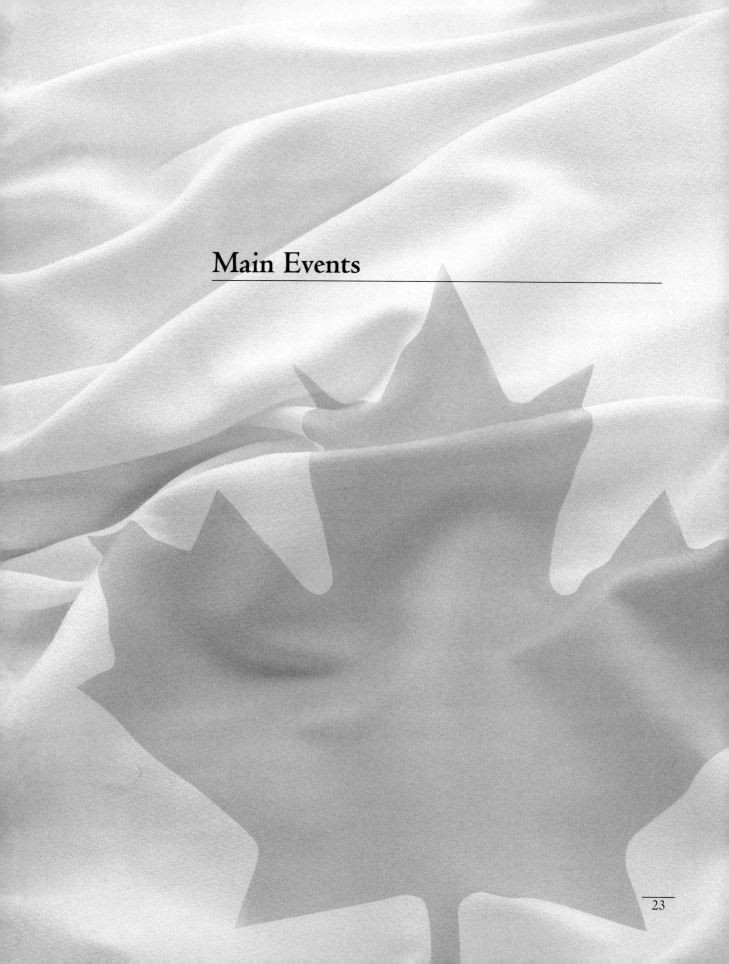

Main Events

Beef Stroganoff

Preparation time: 30 minutes

This is Nancy's favourite recipe because it is an excellent source of protein and iron. It's easy to prepare and is just as good the next day as leftovers. She normally eats it for dinner after training. Her mother used to make it when Nancy was younger, so it reminds her of home.

1½ lbs.	boneless sirloin steak, trimmed and cut into ½-inch (6 mm) strips	750 g
I	medium onion, sliced	I
2 Tbsp.	all-purpose flour	25 mL
10-oz. can	condensed beef bouillon	284 mL
½ tsp.	dry mustard	2 mL
2 Tbsp.	tomato paste	25 mL
I Tbsp.	Worcestershire sauce	15 mL
½ cup	plain yogurt or low-fat sour cream	125 mL
10-oz. can	sliced mushrooms	284 mL
¼ cup	chopped fresh parsley	50 mL

In a large nonstick frying pan, sauté beef over medium heat until browned. Add onion, and cook until tender. Remove from pan, reserving pan juices. Blend flour with beef bouillon, and add to pan juices. Add mustard, tomato paste and Worcestershire sauce. Cook, stirring constantly, until thickened. Add beef and onions, then blend in yogurt, mushrooms and parsley. Heat through over low heat; do not boil. Serve with rice or whole-wheat noodles and vegetables (snow peas are good with this). Serves 6.

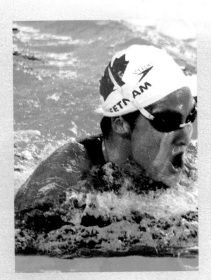

Nancy Sweetnam
S W I M M I N G

A 20-time national champion, Nancy has been on the national swimming team since 1988 and has set nine national and six Commonwealth records in the 200- and 400-metre individual medleys. A partial list of kudos acquired includes being named Canadian Female Swimmer of the Year (1990) and Canadian University Swimmer of the Year (1993). She represented Canada in both the Barcelona and Atlanta Olympic Games.

Nancy is a student at the University of Guelph and a member of the Lightning Bolts Swim Club in Lindsay, Ontario.

Nutritional values per serving
(based on 6 servings):
calories: 216
fat: 7 g; 30% of calories
protein: 29 g; 54% of calories
carbohydrates: 9 g; 16% of calories

Nancy's Performance Eating Tip:

Trim the fat off meats, and use a nonstick pan when cooking.

Mark and John's Healthy Meal

Preparation time: 2½ hours

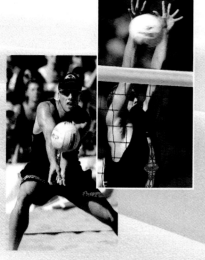

Mark Heese and John Child
B E A C H
V O L L E Y B A L L

Mark and John, both born in Toronto, started competing together in 1995. In 1996, they won the bronze medal in the Olympics, 1st place in the FIVB World Series Tour and the bronze medal in the FIVB world championships. John and Mark rank 1st in Canada and 3rd in the world.

This is John and Mark's favourite peak-performance recipe because it is healthful and can be frozen or set aside for a fast snack when time is short. They usually have it as a snack or lunch on a cold day.

1 lb.	extra-lean ground beef	500 g
1	medium onion, chopped	1
1½ cups	chopped celery	375 mL
1½ cups	chopped carrots	375 mL
1½ cups	chopped potatoes	375 mL
3	beef bouillon cubes	3
48-oz. can	tomato juice	1.36 L
3 cups	water	750 mL
1 cup	pot barley	250 mL

Sauté beef and onion together over medium heat until lightly browned.

Place all ingredients in a large pot, and simmer for 2 hours. Serves 8.

Nutritional values per serving
(based on 8 servings):

calories: 307

fat: 8 g; 24% of calories

protein: 19 g; 25% of calories

carbohydrates: 39 g; 51% of calories

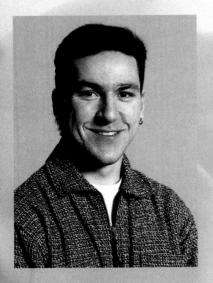

Elvis Stojko's Mom's Burgers

Preparation time: 15 minutes

This is Elvis' favourite recipe because it is tasty and easy to prepare. It provides him with plenty of protein after an intense workout.

1 lb.	ground beef	500 g
1	egg, lightly beaten	1
1	onion, finely chopped	1
⅓ cup	Italian parsley, finely chopped	75 mL
	salt and pepper to taste	
4	hamburger buns, lightly toasted	4

In medium sized bowl, using your hands or fork, combine beef, egg, onion, parsley, salt and pepper until well blended. Form into patties. Barbecue or grill 5 minutes on each side. Split bun in half and fill with burger, adding your own favourite toppings. Serves 4.

Elvis Stojko
MEN'S FIGURE SKATING

Considered by many to be the most technically gifted skater in the world, Elvis possesses the fortitude and tenacity of a true champion. His sparkling career has known many firsts: He was the first ever to land a quadruple toe-double toe loop combination in competition (1991 World Championships) and again took centre stage when he landed the first ever quadruple toe loop-triple toe loop combination at the Champions Series Final in 1997.

Despite a serious injury, Elvis brought home a silver from the Nagano Olympics.

Nutritional values per serving
(based on 4 servings):
calories: 403
fat: 20 g; 46% of calories
protein: 28 g; 28% of calories
carbohydrates: 27 g; 26% of calories

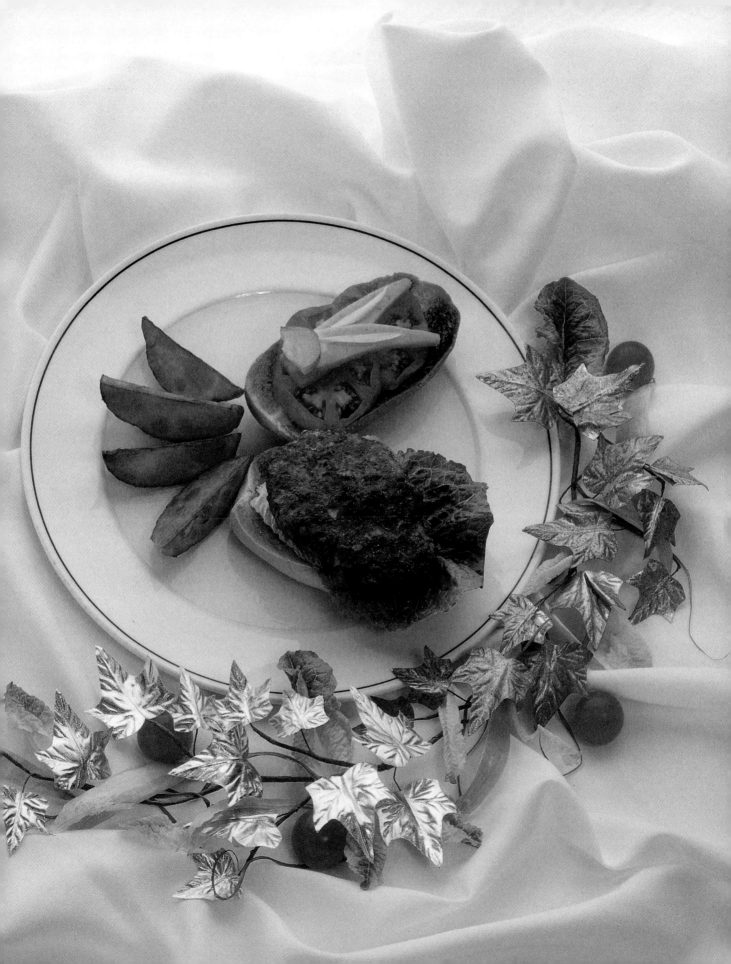

Mama Johl's Burgers

Preparation time: 30 minutes

"There is nothing like a Johl burger to hit the spot. I was raised on them!," says Yogi. This is Yogi's favourite peak-performance lunch, because they are an excellent source of protein.

5 lbs.	lean ground beef	2 kg
2	eggs	2
I	large onion, minced	I
2 Tbsp.	masala	25 mL
½ tsp.	salt	2 mL
½ tsp.	pepper	2 mL
¼ cup	ketchup	50 mL
	whole-wheat buns	
	condiments as desired	

In large bowl, combine onion, egg, spices and ketchup. Add meat, and work mixture into an even texture. Form meat into patties of desired size. Cook on barbecue or on rack in oven with pan to catch drippings. Serve on whole wheat bun with condiments as desired. Serves 12.

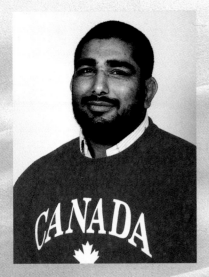

Yogi Johl
WRESTLING

Yogi, a native of Vancouver, British Columbia, is a member of the Burnaby Mountain Wrestling Club. He has been a member of the national team since 1986, and has competed in the NAIA Championships (1995, 1996), the Pan American Championships (1996) and other international competitions. At age 28, he owns and operates his own security company and enjoys playing pool in his spare time.

Nutritional values per serving
(based on 12 servings):
calories: 545
fat: 31 g; 51% of calories
protein: 42 g; 31% of calories
carbohydrates: 24 g; 18% of calories

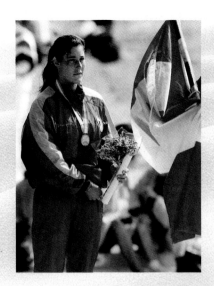

Kelly O'Leary
CANOEING

Kelly, who was born in Halifax and trains at the Cheema Aquatic Club in Waverley, Nova Scotia, has a long string of prizes to her credit. Recent ones include the bronze in the senior K-1 500-metre at the National Championships and silver in the K-2 500-metre at the Pan American Games, both in 1995. In 1996, she was an alternate for the women's kayak team at the Olympics in Atlanta, won silver at the national championships for K-1 500-metre and K-1 200-metre and was selected as Nova Scotia's Female Athlete of the Year.

Nutritional values per serving
(based on 8 servings):
calories: 505
fat: 25 g; 45% of calories
protein: 31 g; 24% of calories
carbohydrates: 38 g; 31% of calories

Sweet and Sour Meatballs With Rice
Preparation time: 1½ hours

Kelly loves this meal, usually after a good workout when she has worked up an appetite. It provides the energy to keep her going.

Meatballs:

2 lbs.	ground beef	I kg
I	small onion, grated	I
2	eggs	2
I tsp.	salt	5 mL
¼ cup	cereal crumbs	50 mL
¼ tsp.	pepper	I mL

Combine all ingredients, and form into 1-inch (2.5 cm) balls. Brown in frying pan. Drain, reserving 2 Tbsp. (25 mL) of pan juices. Arrange meatballs in a casserole dish.

Sweet and Sour Sauce:

14-oz. can	pineapple chunks	398 mL
2 Tbsp.	soy sauce	25 mL
3 Tbsp.	cider vinegar	40 mL
¼ cup	ketchup	50 mL
3 Tbsp.	cornstarch	40 mL
¼ cup	brown sugar	50 mL
½ cup	water	125 mL
I	green pepper, sliced	I
2 Tbsp.	pan juices from meatballs	25 mL

Drain pineapple, reserving juice. Combine pineapple chunks, soy sauce, vinegar, ketchup and cornstarch. Mix well, and pour into frying pan. Add brown sugar and water, and stir until thickened. Add green pepper, pineapple juice and pan juices from meatballs. Pour over meatballs, cover, and bake at 350°F (180°C) for 30 minutes. Serve with rice. Serves 8.

Kelly's Performance Eating Tip:

A healthy diet is especially important if you work out often.

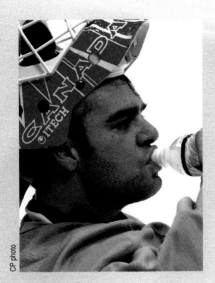

CP photo

Curtis Joseph
H O C K E Y

Originally from Keswick, Ontario, this 31-year-old athlete is currently the goaltender for the Toronto Maple Leafs. He was third in line for the Vezina trophy in 1993, played in the NHL All-Star Game in 1994, and was a member of Team Canada in 1996. Curtis won a silver at the Worlds that same year. He played 71 games in the 1997-98 season and is known for his sportsmanlike conduct and cheerful attitude.

Mushroom Meatloaf

Preparation time: 1 hour

Curtis loves to sit down to this hearty meal after a workout in front of the net. It is easy to prepare and loaded with taste.

1 lb.	lean ground beef	500 g
1	medium egg	1
1 cup	seasoned breadcrumbs	250 mL
¼ cup	table cream	50 g
1	onion, finely diced	1
2 Tbsp.	steak sauce	25 mL
2 tsp.	soy sauce	10 mL
1 cup	chopped mushrooms, sautéed	250 mL
½ cup	grated Swiss cheese	125 mL

Combine all ingredients in a large bowl, and mix thoroughly. Form into a loaf-shaped mound, and place on a lightly greased baking sheet. Bake in preheated 350°F (180°C) oven for 35 minutes or until firm. Let rest for 10 minutes before slicing. Serve with your favourite tomato sauce. Serves 4-6.

Nutritional values per serving
(based on 6 servings without tomato sauce):

calories: 322

fat: 17 g; 47% of calories

protein: 25 g; 31% of calories

carbohydrates: 17 g; 22% of calories

Stuffed Zucchini

Preparation time: 30 minutes

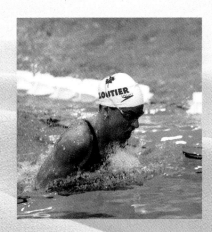

"Meal of champions!" says Guylaine. Ideal before a competition, it is full of vitamins and other nutrients and is easy to digest. She suggests serving it with pasta and sautéed vegetables such as mushrooms, green peppers or onions.

2 Tbsp.	virgin olive oil	25 mL
1 lb.	ground beef or cooked vegetables	500 g
1	large onion, finely chopped	1
1 clove	garlic, chopped	1 clove
1	shallot, finely chopped	1
1	green pepper, finely chopped	1
10-oz. can	tomato sauce	284 mL
pinch	parsley	pinch
	black pepper	
2	medium zucchini, not peeled, cut in half lengthwise	2
½ cup	grated mozzarella cheese	125 mL

Heat 1 Tbsp. (15 mL) olive oil in frying pan, add ground beef, and brown. Remove meat from pan, and set aside. Add the remaining olive oil to the same pan, and sauté onion, garlic, shallot and green pepper. Reduce heat, and return meat to pan. Add tomato sauce, parsley and pepper, and simmer for several minutes. Scoop the flesh out of the zucchini, and fill with meat mixture. Sprinkle mozzarella on top. Place on cookie sheet, and broil for a few minutes until the cheese is browned and bubbling. Serves 4.

Guylaine Cloutier
SWIMMING

Guylaine has been a member of the national swimming team since she was 13 years old. She represented Canada at the 1988, 1992 and 1996 Olympics and was Swimming Canada Female Athlete of the Year in 1992, 1993 and 1995. She has also been selected Quebec Female Swimmer of the Year for a remarkable six years in succession.
  In Seoul in 1988, she was 15th in the 200-metre breaststroke. In Barcelona in 1992, she came 4th in the 100-metre, 5th in the 200-metre and 6th in the 4 x 100 relay. In Atlanta, she placed 5th in the 4 x 100 relay and 6th in the 100-metre breaststroke.

Nutritional values per serving		
(based on 4 servings; with ground beef):		
calories: 417		
fat: 25 g; 55% of calories		
protein: 33 g; 32% of calories		
carbohydrates: 14 g; 13% of calories		

Shannon's Melts

Preparation time: 15 minutes

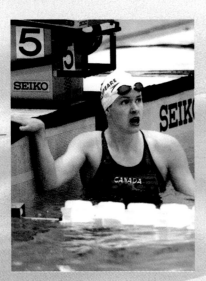

Shannon Shakespeare
SWIMMING

Shannon, Canada's top female sprint freestyle swimmer, is the current Canadian and Commonwealth record holder in the 50-metre freestyle and a seven-time national champion. At the 1996 Canada Cup in Manitoba, she won gold in the 50-metre freestyle and silver in the 100-metre freestyle and 200-metre individual medley.

Shannon usually eats this at lunch or as a balanced snack before a workout. Because it is easy to prepare, it accommodates her busy schedule. A can of shrimp or tuna can be substituted for the bacon and ground beef.

10-oz. can	tomato soup	284 mL
8 slices	bacon, cooked and crumbled	8 slices
½ cup	cooked ground beef	125 mL
1 cup	grated cheddar cheese	250 mL
1	small onion, chopped	1
½ cup	chopped mushrooms	125 mL
1 small	green pepper, chopped	1 small
pinch	garlic salt	pinch
pinch	paprika	pinch
	grated mozzarella cheese	

In a saucepan, combine all ingredients except mozzarella cheese. Heat over low heat until cheese is melted. Spread on as many split buns as there are people to feed, and top with mozzarella. Broil until cheese melts. Refrigerate leftover sauce. Serves 6.

Nutritional values per serving
(based on 6 servings):
calories: 223
fat: 14 g; 58% of calories
protein: 12 g; 22% of calories
carbohydrates: 11 g; 20% of calories

Power-Train Tortellini

Preparation time: 15 minutes

This is Laryssa's favourite meal because it is quick and easy to make with fresh vegetables and pasta. She finds it a perfect pre-event food and normally eats it the night before she competes.

1-lb. pkg.	fresh cheese or meat tortellini	500 g
1 clove	garlic, chopped	1 clove
1	medium onion, chopped	1
1 each	green, red and orange peppers, chopped	1 each
3	medium tomatoes, chopped	3
3	sun-dried tomatoes, chopped	3
¼ cup	feta cheese, crumbled	50 mL

Cook tortellini in boiling water according to package directions. Meanwhile, sauté garlic and onions in a frying pan over medium heat. When they are tender, add peppers, fresh tomatoes and sun-dried tomatoes. Drain tortellini, and place in a large bowl. Add vegetable mixture and feta cheese, stir and serve. Serves 4.

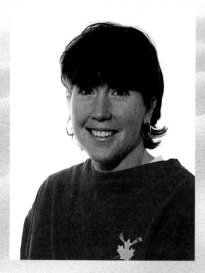

Laryssa Biesenthal
R O W I N G

Laryssa began rowing in 1990 in the University of British Columbia novice rowing program. In 1994, her team won silver in the women's 4x at the Commonwealth Regatta. At the world rowing championships in 1995, they again won silver, and in 1996, they came away from Atlanta with a bronze. Laryssa is currently an interior design student at the Pacific Academy of Design in Victoria.

Nutritional values per serving
(based on 4 servings):
calories: 441
fat: 10 g; 21% of calories
protein: 21 g; 19% of calories
carbohydrates: 67 g; 60% of calories

Spaghetti With Meat Sauce

Preparation time: 30-45 minutes

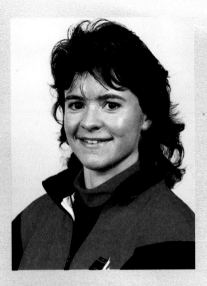

Karen Doell
S O F T B A L L

Karen's hometown is Winkler, Manitoba, where she is a physiotherapist at a sports-injury clinic. When she was growing up, she spent a lot of time playing baseball, street hockey and any sport she could get into. On her first out-of-province trip with a little-league all-star team to Lethbridge, Alberta, she realized that softball was not only a lot of fun but also held some potential for her.

"I had always dreamed of playing softball at the highest possible level. Atlanta in 1996 was the best experience of my life. We had a team with heart and unity—proud to represent Canada. It was my dream come true."

This is Karen's favourite peak-performance recipe because it is quick and easy and provides great carbohydrates. "It tastes fantastic," she says. She usually eats this for supper before a game.

1 lb.	lean ground beef	500 g
28-oz. can	stewed tomatoes	796 mL
10-oz. can	tomato soup	284 mL
5½-oz. can	tomato paste	156 mL
½ cup	water	125 mL
1	medium onion, chopped	1
10 oz.	mushrooms	300 g
½	green pepper, chopped	½
2 Tbsp.	brown sugar	25 mL
1 tsp.	basil	5 mL
2 tsp.	oregano	10 mL
	garlic salt	
2	bay leaves	2
1 lb.	uncooked spaghetti	500 g

Brown beef, and drain off fat. Stir in all other ingredients except spaghetti. Bring to a boil, reduce heat, and simmer for 15 minutes. Meanwhile, cook spaghetti in boiling water and drain. Serve sauce over spaghetti. Serves 6-8.

Nutritional values per serving
(based on 8 servings):
calories: 433
fat: 10 g; 20% of calories
protein: 24 g; 23% of calories
carbohydrates: 62 g; 57% of calories

Manicotti Parmigiana

Preparation time: 1½ hours

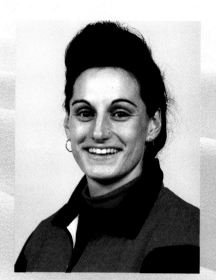

Carmie Vairo
S O F T B A L L

Carmie has been a quiet leader on the Canadian Women's Softball Team since she became a member three years ago. She plays predominantly 2nd base and is an excellent hitter with great base-running speed. She played at the 1995 Pan American Games in Argentina and was also a member of the team that travelled to Guatemala for the Pan American qualifications.

Carmie was raised in Surrey, British Columbia, and now resides in Vancouver.

Carmie usually eats this dish after a competition.

½ lb.	manicotti	250 g
1½ lbs.	ground beef	750 g
½ tsp.	garlic powder	2 mL
½ cup	mushrooms, chopped	125 mL
½	green pepper, finely chopped	½
3 slices	whole-wheat bread, crumbled	3 slices
¾ cup	skim milk	150 mL
2 cups	grated mozzarella cheese	500 mL
1 tsp.	salt	5 mL
¼ tsp.	pepper	1 mL
1 tsp.	chili powder	5 mL
1	egg, lightly beaten	1
28-oz. can	spaghetti sauce	796 mL
½ cup	grated Parmesan cheese	125 mL

Bring a large pot of salted water to a boil. Add half the manicotti, cook for 5 minutes, drain, and set aside. Repeat with remaining shells. Season ground beef with garlic powder, and brown in frying pan. Add mushrooms and green pepper, and sauté until tender. Drain meat, and set aside. Soak breadcrumbs in milk, then add mozzarella, salt, pepper and chili powder. Combine with ground beef mixture. Add egg, and mix well. Stuff mixture into manicotti shells.

Spread half the spaghetti sauce in bottom of a large shallow baking dish. Arrange manicotti in a single layer, and cover with remaining spaghetti sauce. Sprinkle with grated Parmesan cheese. Cover dish with foil, and bake at 350°F (180°C) for 45 minutes. Serves 6-8.

Carmie's Performance Tip:

Get plenty of sleep and exercise to relieve the stress of daily routines.

Nutritional values per serving
(based on 8 servings):
calories: 521
fat: 24 g; 42% of calories
protein: 37 g; 28% of calories
carbohydrates: 39 g; 30% of calories

Beefy Macaroni Skillet

Preparation time: 25 minutes

This is a great quick meal, easy to prepare, easy to eat, easy to clean up after. Perfect for athletes who love to cook but hate to clean up!

1 lb.	extra-lean ground beef	500 g
1	medium onion, chopped	1
1 can	condensed Italian-style tomato soup	1 can
½ cup	water	125 mL
3 Tbsp.	Worcestershire sauce	40 mL
½ cup	marble cheese, shredded	125 mL
2 cups	fusilli or other noodle	500 mL
	black pepper, cayenne pepper and paprika to taste	

In a medium-to-large skillet, over medium-high heat, fry beef and onion until brown, stirring frequently. Pour off any fat. Add soup, water, Worcestershire, and seasonings. Cook pasta until tender. Mix pasta with beef mixture, and top with grated cheese. Serve with garlic toast. Serves 4.

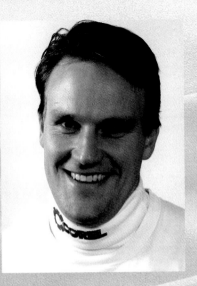

Pierre Lueders
B O B S L E I G H

Despite a relatively late start in the sport, Pierre has enjoyed a stunning career. In 1992, he became the only driver ever to win a gold medal in his very first World Cup race. He was an avid participant in high school track and field, but on the advice of his German cousin, Pierre began working with the Alberta Bobsled Association. He has since competed in the 1996 and 1997 World Championships, and the 1994 and 1998 Olympics.

Nutritional values per serving
(based on 4 servings):
calories: 519
fat: 21 g; 36% of calories
protein: 38 g; 30% of calories
carbohydrates: 44 g; 34% of calories

Floor-Routine Pasta

Preparation time: 20-30 minutes

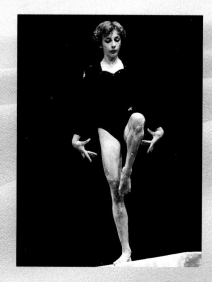

Yvonne Tousek
G Y M N A S T I C S

Yvonne lives with her family in Cambridge, Ontario. At age 12, she was the Canadian Novice Champion and placed 3rd in the youth Pan American Games in Brazil. She has represented Canada at two world championships and was 1995 Canadian Gymnastics Federation Athlete of the Year. At the 1996 Olympics, she was the only Canadian to advance into the individual finals, finishing 26th all-around.

Yvonne says this is her favourite meal because it's simple to make, it's light yet filling and nutritious, and it gives her energy. She eats it for lunch just before training or the night before a meet.

4 cups	uncooked pasta (any kind)	1 L
3 Tbsp.	salt	40 mL
1	large onion, chopped	1
1 lb.	cooked ham, cut into small pieces	500 g
¼ cup	vegetable oil	50 mL
1 cup	corn	250 mL
1 cup	peas	250 mL
1 cup	fresh green beans, sliced	250 mL
⅓ cup	chives, finely chopped	75 mL

Bring a large pot of water to a boil. Add pasta and 2 Tbsp. (25 mL) of the salt, and cook for 12-14 minutes. Drain, rinse, and set aside. In a frying pan over medium heat, sauté onion and ham in oil for about 3 minutes. Blanch corn, peas and green beans in boiling water and remaining salt for about 2 minutes, then drain. Combine all ingredients in a large serving dish, sprinkle with chives, and serve. Serves 4-6.

Nutritional values per serving
(based on 6 servings):
calories: 368
fat: 15 g; 37% of calories
protein: 20 g; 21% of calories
carbohydrates: 38 g; 42% of calories

Points-Race Pizza

Preparation time: 1½ hours

This is one of Brian's favourite meals because it tastes good and fills him up but is not too heavy. He eats it as a snack in the evening or as the main course for dinner.

I cup	tomato paste or pasta sauce	250 mL
	Tomato-Basil Thin Pizza Crust (see below)	
I	small onion, sliced	I
8 oz.	spicy pepperoni	250 g
I	medium red pepper, cubed	I
14-oz.can	pineapple chunks, drained	398 mL
I	medium tomato, thinly sliced, seeds removed	I
6-8	mushrooms	6-8
½ cup	tofu	125 mL
½ cup	Parmesan cheese	125 mL

Preheat oven to 450°F (230°C). Spread tomato paste on the pizza crust. Arrange all remaining ingredients on top, finishing off with Parmesan cheese. Place on upper rack of the oven, and cook for 10-15 minutes.

Tomato-Basil Thin Pizza Crust:

2 tsp.	active dry yeast	10 mL
I cup	tomato pesto sauce	250 mL
3 Tbsp.	olive oil	40 mL
2 Tbsp.	basil	25 mL
½ tsp.	salt	2 mL
4 cups	flour	I L

Combine yeast and tomato pesto sauce in a medium bowl. Let sit for 2 minutes. Add olive oil. In another bowl, mix basil, salt and flour. Slowly mix the dry ingredients into the yeast mixture until dough becomes stiff. Knead on a lightly floured surface for 5-10 minutes. Place dough in a greased bowl, cover, and let rise for 45 minutes to I hour. Form dough into a pizza crust on a large greased pizza pan. Serves 6-8.

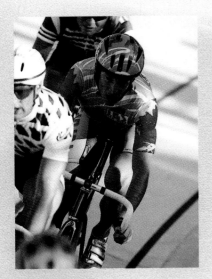

Brian Walton
CYCLING

Brian is a leader on the Canadian cycling team. He was a member of the 1988 and 1996 Olympic teams and has competed and won medals in the Commonwealth and Pan American Games. In Atlanta, he won silver in the points race. Brian has been racing on the professional circuit for the past eight years and is currently riding for the Saturn racing team.

Nutritional values per serving
(based on 8 servings):
calories: 565
fat: 23 g; 36% of calories
protein: 19 g; 14% of calories
carbohydrates: 71 g; 50% of calories

Chicken Cacciatore

Preparation time: 5 hours

Kelly usually eats this the evening prior to competition. She says this recipe has an "awesome taste with egg noodles."

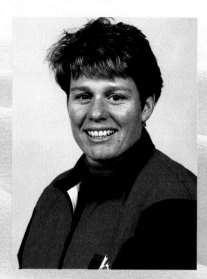

Kelly Kelland
S O F T B A L L

Kelly was a member of Canada's national softball team from 1986 to 1996. Her career highlights include three Pan American Games, two world championships and, most recently, the Olympic Games in Atlanta. She officially retired from the national team after the Olympics and was awarded Senior Softball Athlete of the Year for British Columbia. Kelly is 34 years old and resides in Kamloops, British Columbia, where she is a child- and youth-care counsellor. In her spare time, she enjoys fishing, camping, exercising and especially rollerblading.

3 cloves	garlic, chopped	3 cloves
1	large onion, chopped	1
1 Tbsp.	vegetable oil	15 mL
1	whole chicken	1
14-oz. can	tomato sauce	398 mL
2 5½-oz. cans	tomato paste	312 mL
48-oz. can	tomato juice	1.36 L can
2 10-oz. cans	mushrooms	568 mL
1	bay leaf	1
½ tsp.	celery seeds	2 mL
½ tsp.	basil	2 mL
½ tsp.	pepper	2 mL
2 tsp.	oregano	10 mL
	fresh parsley	

In a large pot, sauté garlic and onion in oil. Add chicken, then boiling water to cover. Simmer for 30 minutes. Remove chicken from heat, allow to cool, and remove skin and bones. Return to pot. Add tomato sauce, tomato paste and tomato juice. Stir, then add remaining ingredients. Simmer for 4-5 hours. Serves 6-8.

Nutritional values per serving
(based on 6 servings):
calories: 298
fat: 5 g; 15% of calories
protein: 31 g; 41% of calories
carbohydrates: 33 g; 44% of calories

Oriental Chicken Wings

Preparation time: 1 hour

"*This meal tastes terrific," says Keith, "and it can be enjoyed for more than one meal — it's good heated up for a quick lunch. A 3:1 ratio of rice to wings gives you high carbohydrates and protein in the proper proportion. You can eat it before or after an event, and while it is not the ultimate dieting food, it is great after a weigh-in or a competition." In Keith's opinion, the best rice is Japanese (Kokoho Rose), prepared in a rice cooker.*

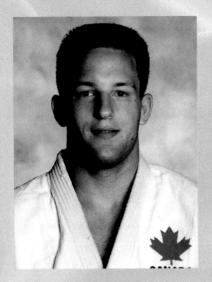

3 lbs.	chicken wings	1.5 kg
1	egg, lightly beaten	1
1 cup	flour	250 mL
1 cup	butter	250 mL
3 Tbsp.	soy sauce	40 mL
½ cup	vinegar	125 mL
3 Tbsp.	water	40 mL
1 tsp.	seasoned salt	5 mL
¾ cup	white sugar	150 mL
½ tsp.	salt	2 mL
1½ cups	rice	375 mL

Dip wings in egg, then flour. In a frying pan, cook in butter over medium heat until browned and crisp. Meanwhile, combine remaining ingredients in a small bowl to make sauce. Place wings in shallow roasting pan, and pour sauce over them. Bake at 350°F (180°C) for 30 minutes. Spoon sauce over wings a few times during cooking. Cook rice while wings are in oven. Leftover wings taste good heated up the next day. Serves 6.

Keith Morgan
J U D O

Keith, who has been practising judo for 16 years and has a 3rd-degree black belt, is a member of the Canadian Olympic judo team (95-kg class). He was a two-time Canadian junior champion and has been senior champion (95-kg) for the past three years. Keith placed in the top 16 at the 1996 Olympics and has also earned several international titles, including the gold in the 1995 Pan American Games. Keith is a Petro-Canada OlympicTorch Scholarship recipient.

Nutritional values per serving
(based on 6 servings):
calories: 1124
fat: 65 g; 52% of calories
protein: 53 g; 19% of calories
carbohydrates: 81 g; 29% of calories

Keith's Performance Eating Tip:

"*I tend to shy away from ready-to-serve meals because you can never be sure what you are eating. Your own creations, made with fresh ingredients, are not only satisfying but fun too.*"

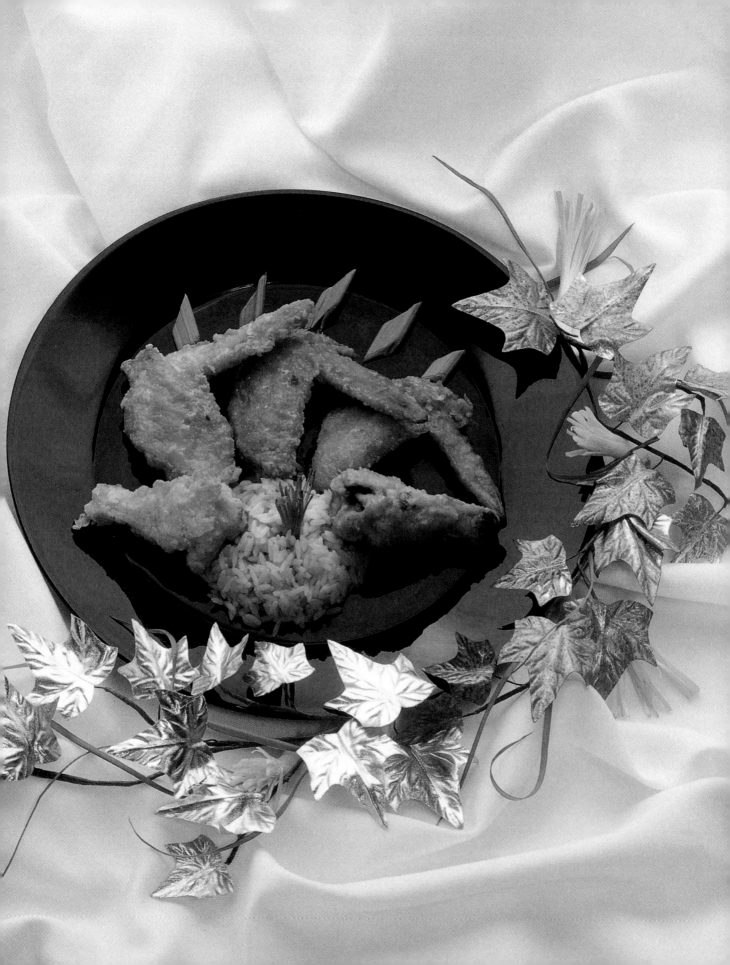

Chicken Chili

Preparation time: 45 minutes

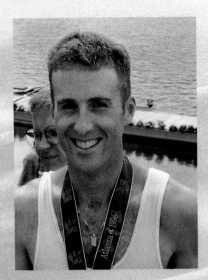

Jeff Lay
R O W I N G

Jeff is a member of the lightweight 4s, which took a silver medal in an impressive showing at the 1996 Olympics. Jeff is a single-minded, committed competitor, and since entering the sport some ten years ago, he has been building an enviable record in the world of international rowing. In 1996, his squad took a bronze medal in the Lucerne Rotsee Regatta and a gold at the Duisberg Regatta in Germany. These can be added to his gold medal in the 1995 U.S. nationals and many other achievements. Jeff is now the varsity rowing coach at the University of Western Ontario.

Jeff finds Chicken Chili easy to make, tasty and healthful. He also likes it because there is always some left over for lunch the next day. He usually eats it at dinner or lunch during winter training in off-season.

¾ lb.	ground chicken	375 g
1 cup	chopped onions	250 mL
½ cup	chopped green pepper	125 mL
2 cloves	garlic, minced	2 cloves
14-oz.	can tomatoes	398 mL
19-oz.	can dark red kidney beans	540 mL
1 cup	sliced mushrooms	250 mL
8-oz. can	tomato sauce	213 mL
2-3 tsp.	chili powder	10-15 mL
½ tsp.	crushed basil	2 mL
¼ tsp.	salt	1 mL
¼ tsp.	pepper	1 mL

In a large saucepan, cook chicken, onions, pepper and garlic until meat is brown. Drain off fat. Add tomatoes, cutting them up, then stir in remaining ingredients and bring to a boil. Reduce heat, cover, and simmer for 20 minutes, stirring occasionally. Serves 4.

Nutritional values per serving
(based on 4 servings):
calories: 291
fat: 8 g; 24% of calories
protein: 19 g; 27% of calories
carbohydrates: 36 g; 50% of calories

Finish-Line Chicken

Preparation time: 15-20 minutes

This is Janice's favourite recipe because it is an absolutely delicious balanced meal. It's a recipe her mom made for her on special occasions, and now she prepares it when she wants to spoil herself and her family. When served with rice and veggies, it provides a good balance of protein and carbohydrates. She eats it after hard mental and physical work. The protein recharges muscles and brain. Janice feels that nutrition is the most difficult area to make changes in because it is so easy to get hooked on "undesirable" foods.

1½ lbs.	chicken breasts, boned, skinned and cut up	750 g
1	medium onion, chopped	1
1 cup	ketchup	250 mL
⅓ cup	water	75 mL
¼ cup	sherry	50 mL
1 Tbsp.	Worcestershire sauce	15 mL
2 Tbsp.	margarine	25 mL
2 Tbsp.	lemon juice	25 mL
1 Tbsp.	brown sugar	15 mL

Place chicken in casserole dish. Cover, and cook in microwave for 5 minutes on medium. Combine remaining ingredients in separate bowl, and pour over chicken. Return to microwave, and cook, covered, on medium for 8-10 minutes. Serve with rice and veggies on the side. Serves 4.

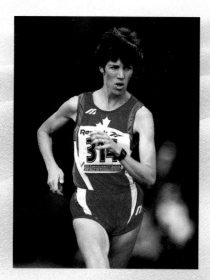

Janice McCaffrey
R A C E W A L K I N G

Over a decade ago, Janice transformed herself from an avid runner into a world-class racewalker. In 1992 and 1996, her efforts were rewarded when she competed for Canada at the Barcelona and Atlanta Olympic Games. Janice's quest for the year 2000 is to compete, at 40, in her 3rd Olympic Games.

Janice has won nine Canadian titles in racewalking. At the 1994 Commonwealth Games, she was the first Canadian ever to win a medal in the 10-km event. She won a gold medal at the 1994 Francophone Games and three U.S. championships. She is also a Pan American Games Racewalk Cup silver medallist.

Nutritional values per serving
(based on 4 servings):
calories: 385
fat: 11 g; 25% of calories
protein: 44 g; 46% of calories
carbohydrates: 24 g; 25% of calories

Janice's Performance Eating Tip:

Set goals, and challenge yourself to learn about eating for peak performance. As with training, it takes commitment and patience to make positive changes. It's worth it, and it can be very tasty too!

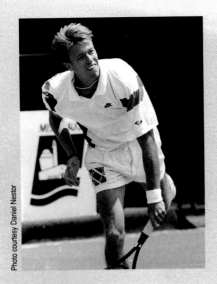

Daniel Nestor
T E N N I S

Daniel began playing tennis when he was eight years old. He has been a member of Canada's Davis Cup team since 1990 and is one of the country's most recognizable players. A member of the world-champion Canadian Sunshine Cup team in 1989 (runners-up in 1990), he is ranked number three in the world (with partner Mark Knowles) in doubles.

Chicken Tortillas

Preparation time: 30 minutes

"These tortillas," says Daniel, "are high in fibre, calcium, protein and carbohydrates and are an excellent source of iron. This is my favourite meal (dinner) before a competition."

1 lb.	chicken breasts, boned and skinned	500 g
3 Tbsp.	olive oil	40 mL
1 Tbsp.	chili powder	15 mL
1	onion, sliced	1
1	banana pepper, sliced	1
1 each	green and red peppers, sliced	1 each
1	zucchini, sliced lengthwise	1
	salt and pepper	
3 Tbsp.	lime juice	40 mL
1 clove	garlic, minced	1 clove
4	10-inch (25 cm) flour tortillas	4
½ cup	sour cream or salsa	125 mL

Slice chicken into thin strips. Combine 1 Tbsp. oil with chili powder, and toss with chicken. In a large frying pan, heat remaining oil, add chicken, and cook, stirring, for about 5 minutes. Remove, and set aside. In the same pan, cook onion, banana pepper, red and green peppers and zucchini for 8 minutes. Return chicken to pan, season with salt and pepper to taste, and cook until heated through. Add lime juice and garlic. Meanwhile, wrap tortillas in foil, and warm them in a 350°F (180°C) oven for 3 minutes. Place chicken mixture in tortillas with sour cream or salsa. Serves 4.

Nutritional values per serving
(based on 4 servings; with sour cream):
calories: 471
fat: 22 g; 43% of calories
protein: 35 g; 30% of calories
carbohydrates: 32 g; 28% of calories

Aristotle Chicken

Preparation time: 10 minutes or 1¼ hours depending on cooking method.

Therese says that this is her favourite way to prepare chicken, because it is healthy, quick, and tastes great when cooked on the barbecue.

4	skinned chicken breasts	4
2 cups	no-fat mayonnaise	500 mL
4 Tbsp.	honey	50 mL
6 Tbsp.	Dijon style honey mustard	75 mL
2 tsp.	Worcestershire sauce	10 mL
1 tsp.	lemon juice	5 mL
	herbs and spices to taste	

Preheat barbecue or oven to 350°F (180°C). Whisk together mayonnaise, honey, mustard, Worcestershire sauce and lemon juice until well blended. Dip chicken into mixture. If grilling, shake on desired seasonings and grill for 2-3 minutes on each side. If baking, place dipped pieces of chicken on large sheet of foil, pour sauce over it, and fold foil around chicken to form a seal. Bake for 60 minutes, remove from foil, then shake on desired seasonings to garnish. Serves 4.

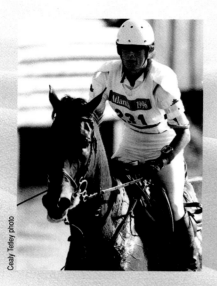

Cealy Tettey photo

Therese Washtock
E Q U E S T R I A N

Even as a little girl, Therese dreamed of one day competing in the Olympics and has been a member of the national team since the age of 16. Her achievements include: BC Award of Excellence (five times), High Point BC Rider Award (eight years), and in 1995 ranked fifth in North America in the FEI Landrover World Rankings. While continuing to compete, she operates Quail Crossing Farm in Summerland, British Columbia, and enjoys tutoring others in equestrian pursuits.

Nutritional values per serving *(based on 4 servings):*
calories: 678
fat: 31 g; 41% of calories
protein: 60 g; 35% of calories
carbohydrates: 40 g; 24% of calories

Therese's Performance Eating Tip:

Stick to low-fat substitutes, and you will find that your taste buds adjust over time. Drink plenty of water!

Cajun Chicken Jambalaya

Preparation time: 45 minutes

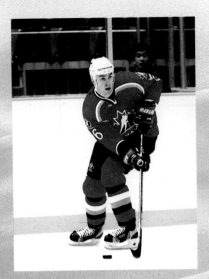

Trevor Linden
HOCKEY

Trevor, who stands 6'4" without skates, was Vancouver's first choice in the 1988 draft. Ten years later, he boasts many fine accomplishments. He has played on the Memorial Cup All-Star team, the NHL All-Rookie team, and the NHL All-Star Team. Trevor won the King Clancy Memorial Trophy in 1996-97. He has been referred to as a "gritty power forward," and is known for pulling out all the stops when it really counts.

Trevor loves this meal because of its wonderful blend of flavours—it is truly "variety on a plate!"

8	slices bacon, diced	8
I	whole medium-size chicken, cut into 8 pieces	I
I½	cups long-diced Black Forest ham	375 mL
I	large onion, diced	I
2 cloves	garlic	2 cloves
2 cups	long-grain rice	500 mL
2½ cups	hot chicken stock	625 mL
I lb.	tomatoes, peeled, seeded and diced	500 g
2 tsp.	salt	10 mL
I tsp.	Tabasco sauce	5 mL
I lb.	baby shrimp	500 g
	fresh dill, chopped	

In a hot frying pan, cook bacon until crisp, then remove from pan. In the bacon fat, cook chicken pieces until browned, then remove from pan. Brown ham, onions and garlic in the same oil. Add rice, and stir until coated with fat. Add chicken stock, tomatoes and seasonings, and bring to a boil. Add chicken, shrimp, and bacon and cover. Bring back to a boil, and place in a preheated 350°F (180°C) oven for 18 minutes or until liquid is absorbed. Arrange on platter with rice on the bottom and chicken and garnishes on top. Sprinkle with fresh dill. Serves 8.

Nutritional values per serving
(based on 8 servings):
calories: 388
fat: 10 g; 23% of calories
protein: 31 g; 31% of calories
carbohydrates: 44 g; 46% of calories

Chicken Parmesan

Preparation time: 30 minutes

This is Chris's favourite peak-performance meal. It's quick and easy to prepare and packed with taste.

4	chicken breasts, boned, skinned and flattened	4
2	eggs, beaten	2
I cup	breadcrumbs seasoned with salt and pepper	250 mL
2 Tbsp.	butter	25 mL
I cup	canned tomato sauce	250 mL
I cup	shredded low-fat mozzarella	250 mL
I tsp.	grated Parmesan cheese	5 mL
2 Tbsp.	chopped fresh basil	25 mL
2 Tbsp.	chopped fresh parsley	25 mL

Dip chicken breasts into eggs and then into breadcrumbs, making sure the chicken is evenly coated. Heat butter in a medium skillet, and gently brown chicken breasts on both sides. Place on a baking sheet in preheated 350°F (180°C) oven for 8-10 minutes. Meanwhile, heat tomato sauce. When chicken is done, pour sauce over it, then sprinkle cheeses and herbs on top. Return to oven for a few minutes until cheese is melted. Serves 4.

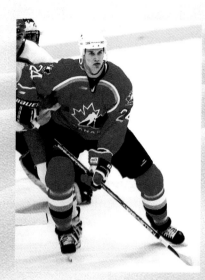

Chris Pronger
H O C K E Y

Standing 6'5" and weighing in at 220 pounds, Chris is clearly built to be a strong defenceman. Chris played 81 games with the St. Louis Blues in the 1997-98 season, and is known for his excellent skating ability.

Chris is a native of Dryden, Ontario, and was the Hartford Whalers' first choice in the 1993 draft, the same year he played in the Junior Worlds. He was a member of the NHL All-Rookie team in 1994.

Nutritional values per serving
(based on 4 servings):
calories: 578
fat: 21 g; 33% of calories
protein: 73g; 51% of calories
carbohydrates: 24g; 17% of calories

Lemon-Mustard Chicken Breasts Over Basmati Rice

Preparation time: 1 hour

This is May's favourite peak-performance recipe because the rice provides the complex carbohydrates needed for endurance running and there's just enough fat in the chicken to leave her feeling satisfied the night before a race.

4	chicken breasts, boned and skinned	4
2 Tbsp.	minced green onion	25 mL
1 Tbsp.	vegetable oil	15 mL
1 Tbsp.	lemon juice	15 mL
1 tsp.	Worcestershire sauce	5 mL
2 Tbsp.	Dijon mustard	25 mL
pinch	salt and pepper	pinch
1½ cups	basmati rice	375 mL
2 cups	water	500 mL
	oil	
	salt	

Place chicken in deep baking dish. Combine onion, 1 Tbsp. oil, lemon juice, Worcestershire sauce and mustard in a bowl, mix thoroughly, and pour over chicken. Cover, and bake at 375°F (190°C) for 45 minutes. Meanwhile, place rice in nonstick saucepan, pour water over it, and add oil and salt to taste. Cook, uncovered, on high heat until all water is absorbed. Reduce heat to low, cover pot with paper towel and lid, and let stand for 15 minutes. Serve chicken over rice. Serves 4.

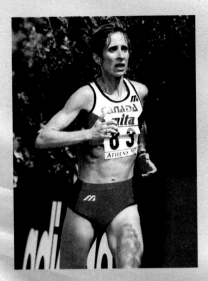

May Allison
RUNNING

May has been on the Canadian national team since 1984. She has an H.B.A. from the University of Western Ontario and was Western's Female Athlete of the Year in 1987. In 1996, she competed in the Olympics, won the Columbia 10-km and came in 2nd in the Cleveland Marathon. Since graduating from university, she has competed on several national teams and raced well at various distances. Recently, she has concentrated her efforts on the marathon and successfully earned a spot on the 1996 Canadian Olympic team.

Nutritional values per serving
(based on 4 servings):
calories: 446
fat: 8 g; 16% of calories
protein: 35 g; 31% of calories
carbohydrates: 60 g; 53% of calories

May's Performance Eating Tip:

Variety is the spice of life!

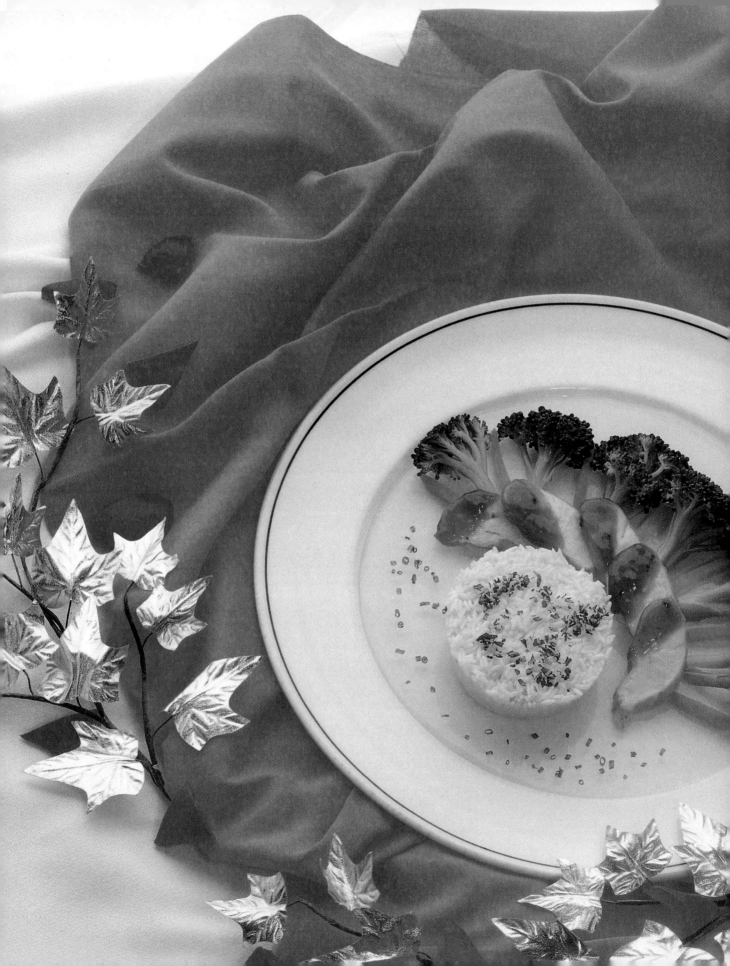

HANNAM STOREY

Paul Hannam and Brian Storey
Y A C H T I N G

Paul and Brian, both 25, sailed together for more than nine years before being selected to compete in the 1996 Olympics. Their search for training sites and regattas has led them to locations as diverse as San Francisco, Helsinki and Wabamun, Alberta. Often, their trips entail camping and cooking over a portable propane stove or campfire, the origin of this recipe. Brian, who is engaged to be married, works in Washington, D.C., and Paul, recently married, attends university in Vancouver.

Hearty Campfire Chicken Dinner

Preparation time: 2½ hours

Paul and Brian say this is their favourite peak-performance recipe because it can be cooked in one pot over a propane stove or a campfire. It tastes wonderful, fills you up and is full of protein and trace minerals. They normally eat this following a long day on the water, when they need to replace energy but want something with more flavour than pasta.

4	chicken breasts, boned, skinned and sliced	4
I	medium potato, diced	I
I Tbsp.	oil	15 mL
I	large onion, diced	I
8-10	mushrooms, quartered	8-10
I	green pepper, diced	I
2 cups	plain yogurt	500 mL
6 Tbsp.	tomato paste	75 mL
½	lime, juice and pulp	½
I-2 Tbsp.	curry powder or paste	15-25 mL

In a large covered pot, cook chicken and potato in oil over medium heat (about 10 minutes). Add onion, and cook 2 minutes, then add mushrooms, green pepper, yogurt, tomato paste and curry powder to taste. Reduce heat, and cook, covered, for up to 2 hours. It tastes better the longer you leave it. Serve over rice. Serves 3-4 people, depending on appetites.

Nutritional values per serving
(based on 4 servings; without rice):
calories: 378
fat: 12 g; 27% of calories
protein: 37 g; 39% of calories
carbohydrates: 31 g; 33% of calories

Chicken and Vegetable Rolls

Preparation time: 45 minutes

Chris says this dish goes well with steamed vegetables and rice. A complete peak-performance meal!

2	garlic cloves, chopped	2
⅔ cup	fresh spinach, chopped	150 mL
⅓ cup	fresh coriander, chopped	75 mL
¼ cup	Dijon mustard	50 mL
¼ cup	yogurt	50 mL
½ tsp.	salt	2 mL
½ tsp.	ground black pepper	2 mL
I tsp.	lemon juice	5 mL
4	skinless, boneless chicken breasts	4
6 slices	Emmenthal (Swiss) cheese	6 slices
4 thin slices	Black Forest ham	4 thin slices
4 slices	lemon	4 slices

Preheat oven to 375°F (190°C). In a bowl, combine garlic, spinach, coriander, mustard, yogurt, salt, pepper, and I tsp. of the lemon juice. Stir until well blended. Gently pound chicken breasts flat. Spread sauce on uneven side of chicken. Top each breast with a slice of cheese, then a slice of ham. Cut remaining slices of cheese in half and set aside. Gently roll up chicken, securing each with a toothpick. Arrange in a non-stick baking dish and top each breast with half a slice of cheese and a slice of lemon. Bake for 20-25 minutes. Sprinkle with pepper and lemon juice, and serve immediately. Serves 4.

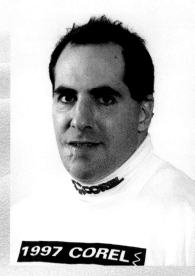

Chris Lori
B O B S L E I G H

A member of the national team since 1985, Chris has competed in four Olympic Games, and numerous World Championships. He is a native of Windsor, Ontario, and is a member of the Ontario Bobsleigh Association. Chris now resides in Vancouver, British Columbia, and enjoys windsurfing, hockey, tennis, golf and reading.

Nutritional values per serving
(based on 4 servings):

calories: 693

fat: 25 g; 33% of calories

protein: 70 g; 41% of calories

carbohydrates: 46 g; 27% of calories

Slider Chicken Delight (Stir-Fry)

Preparation time: 40 minutes

This is Christine's favourite recipe because it provides protein and carbohydrates (two important ingredients for muscle power and refuelling) without a lot of fat. She normally eats this dish prior to game day to allow time for proper digestion.

4	chicken breasts, boned and skinned	4
1 tsp.	sesame seeds	5 mL
4 tsp.	red wine vinegar	20 mL
4 tsp.	light soy sauce	20 mL
4 tsp.	sesame oil	20 mL
1 Tbsp.	grated fresh ginger	15 mL
2 cloves	garlic, crushed	2 cloves
½ tsp.	sugar	2 mL
1 tsp.	vegetable oil	5 mL
8 oz.	mushrooms, sliced	250 g
4 cups	red cabbage, grated	1 L
4 oz.	snow peas	125 g
2 cups	cooked rice	500 mL

Rinse chicken, pat dry, and sprinkle with sesame seeds. Cook in a non-stick frying pan over medium-low heat until browned, 12-15 minutes, and set aside. Meanwhile, in a small bowl, stir together vinegar, soy sauce, sesame oil, ginger, garlic and sugar. Heat vegetable oil in a nonstick pan, add mushrooms, and stir-fry for 3 minutes. Add cabbage, and stir-fry for 2 minutes. Add snow peas, and cook until bright green, about 2 minutes. Add vinegar mixture, and stir for 1 more minute. Cut chicken diagonally across the grain and arrange over vegetables. Serve with rice. Serves 4.

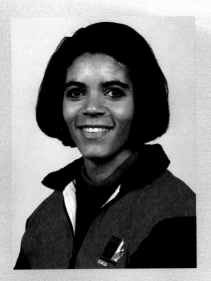

Christine Parris-Washington
S O F T B A L L

Christine joined the Canadian national team in 1991 after compiling a 42-2 pitching record while batting .439 and .407 at the University of Nevada, Las Vegas, and being named Big West Conference Field Player of the Year in 1991. In 1996, she was part of Canada's Olympic squad and the team's athletic representative. At the Canada Cup international tournament, she was named most valuable player. She lives in Las Vegas, Nevada, with her husband Robert.

Nutritional values per serving
(based on 4 servings):
calories: 439
fat: 10 g; 21% of calories
protein: 36 g; 33% of calories
carbohydrates: 50 g; 45% of calories

Christine's Performance Eating Tip:

Diet is as important as physical training. Eating foods that are low in fat is the key to a healthy life.

Japanese Chicken

Preparation time: 50 minutes

Neal enjoys this meal because it is nutritious and tasty. It's a delicious way to warm up after a day spent on the ice.

4	skinless, boneless chicken breasts	4
1 tsp.	garlic salt	5 mL
½ cup	flour	125 mL
2	eggs, beaten	2
2 tsp.	olive oil	10 mL

Preheat oven to 375°F (190°C). Dip chicken in egg, and place in a plastic bag along with the flour and garlic salt to coat. Fry in a nonstick pan with oil. Transfer chicken to a baking pan.

Sauce:

¼ cup	chicken broth	50 mL
¼ cup	vinegar	50 mL
¼ cup	ketchup	50 mL
1 tsp.	soy sauce	5 mL
¾ cup	brown sugar	150 mL
1 tsp.	salt	5 mL

Mix all ingredients in a bowl, then pour over chicken. Bake, uncovered, for 40 minutes. Serves 4.

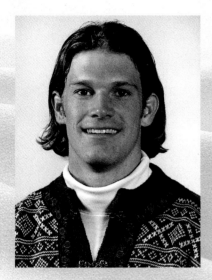

Neal Marshall
SPEED SKATING

The Burnaby Haida Speed Skating Club has good reason to be proud of Neal. He holds the Canadian records in both the 3,000m and 5,000m events. A member of the national team since 1989, Neal has been the Canadian overall champion six years running. When he's not skating with teammates Mike and Kevin (who also happen to be Neal's brothers), he turns his attention to motorcycling.

Nutritional values per serving
(based on 4 servings):

calories: 518

fat: 12 g; 21% of calories

protein: 64 g; 49% of calories

carbohydrates: 39 g; 30% of calories

Chicken à la Curt

Preparation time: 1 hour

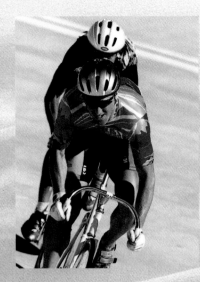

Curt Harnett

C Y C L I N G

Curt began competing in 1981, at the age of 16, and has been a member of the National Team since 1983. He has many first place finishes to his credit, including the World Cup (1996), the Goodwill Games (1990), and is an eight-time Canadian champion who won bronze at Atlanta. Curt was born in Toronto, but currently resides in Thunder Bay, Ontario where he is a member of the "Spirit of Sport" campaign.

"This chicken recipe is a favourite at my house. My wife Treena loves this dish, although my son Skylar still likes my steak over my chicken. I start with as many fresh ingredients as possible - it's the freshness that makes the recipe successful."

6	boneless, skinless chicken breasts	6
6 stems	fresh basil	6 stems
6 cloves	garlic	6 cloves
12	medium tomatoes	12
½ cup	olive oil	125 mL
1 jar	capers	1 jar
¼ cup	red wine	50 mL
1	lemon	1

Preheat oven to 350°F (180°C). Place chicken breasts on a cookie sheet, and lightly brush with oil. Sprinkle with 2-3 crushed garlic cloves and half a squeezed lemon. Slice the other half of the lemon and set aside. Bake chicken for approximately 20 minutes. Remove from oven, top with lemon slices, and bake for an additional 20 minutes.

Sauce Preparation: Blanch and peel the tomatoes. Sauté 2-3 cloves of chopped garlic in a large frying pan with a little olive oil. Add tomatoes, and simmer at a high enough heat for them to begin breaking down quickly. Add chopped basil, red wine, and capers. Simmer for approximately 30 minutes, or until it is a condensed sauce-like consistency.

Place the chicken on a plate and spoon the sauce on top. If desired, serve with a garlic pasta as a side dish.

Nutritional values per serving
(based on 4 servings):
calories: 818
fat: 39 g; 43% of calories
protein: 92 g; 45% of calories
carbohydrates: 22 g; 11% of calories

Ginger Chicken Linguine

Preparation time: 30 minutes

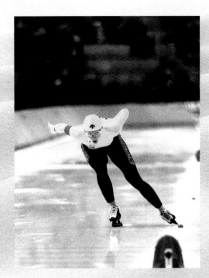

Susan Auch
SPEED SKATING

Susan's career as a speed skater began at age ten, when she watched her brother's power skating class put through its paces by a speed skater. Since then, her love of the sport has brought her many impressive accomplishments. She was the Canadian Amateur Speed Skating Association's female athlete of the year three years in a row (1990-92), and in 1995, was voted TSN's People's Choice for amateur athlete of the year.

  Susan speaks both English and German, and is currently a student at the University of Calgary.

This recipe always reminds me of my first high-altitude training camp. Delia Roberts, the doctor that travelled with us, fed us this meal one evening. Now it is my favourite one to entertain with.

4	boneless, skinless chicken breasts	400 g
1 pkg.	linguine	600 g
2 Tbsp.	gingerroot, chopped	25 mL
6 cloves	garlic, chopped	6 cloves
2 Tbsp.	butter or olive oil	25 mL
1 Tbsp.	fresh basil, chopped	15 mL
1 Tbsp.	fresh cilantro, chopped	15 mL
2 tsp.	hot sauce	10 mL
6	green onions, chopped	6
1 tsp.	ground black pepper	5 mL
½ cup	grated Parmesan cheese	125 mL

Cube the chicken and fry in a skillet. Set aside. In a large pot, cook the linguine. Meanwhile, in a skillet, sauté the ginger and garlic in the butter. Add basil, cilantro, hot sauce, green onions, and pepper. Cook for approximately 2 minutes. Toss together with chicken, linguine, and cheese. Serves 4.

Nutritional values per serving
(based on 4 servings):
calories: 791
fat: 15 g; 17% of calories
protein: 50 g; 25% of calories
carbohydrates: 115 g; 58% of calories

Chicken Fettuccine

Preparation time: 30 minutes

Erminia says this is her favourite peak-performance recipe because it is a quick, easy, all-in-one meal that provides the carbohydrates needed to get through long practices and matches. She usually eats this the night before a match or a big practice day.

I clove	garlic, chopped	I clove
I	small onion, chopped	I
I tsp.	oil	5 mL
2	chicken breasts, boned, skinned and cut into bite-sized pieces	2
¼ tsp.	oregano	I mL
	salt and pepper	
I stalk	celery, sliced	I stalk
I	carrot, sliced	I
I	green pepper, sliced	I
½ cup	sliced mushrooms	125 mL
I cup	2% evaporated milk	250 mL
I	medium tomato, diced	I
3 Tbsp.	Parmesan cheese	40 mL
12 oz.	fettuccine	340 g

In a nonstick frying pan, sauté garlic and onion until softened. Add chicken to pan along with oregano and salt and pepper to taste. Cook until chicken is tender and browned. Add celery, carrot, green pepper and mushrooms, and cook until vegetables are tender. Lower heat, add milk, and cook, stirring, until milk is heated through. Add tomato and Parmesan cheese, cover, and simmer. Meanwhile, in a large pot of boiling water, cook fettuccine until tender. Serve chicken mixture over pasta. Serves 2-4.

Erminia's Performance Eating Tip:

In any recipe, you can substitute evaporated milk for whipping cream or half-and-half to lower calories.

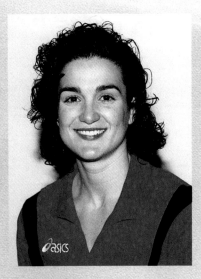

Erminia Russo
VOLLEYBALL

Erminia, who hails from Kelowna, British Columbia, was a member of the 1996 Olympic volleyball team and a member of Team Canada on two occasions. Between 1989 and 1991, she was team captain. She has competed in numerous international tournaments, including the 1986 and 1990 world championships, the World Cup and the Pan American Games. The head coach of the University of British Columbia's women's volleyball team, she lives in Vancouver.

Nutritional values per serving
(based on 4 servings):
calories: 516
fat: 9 g; 15% of calories
protein: 47 g; 36% of calories
carbohydrates: 63 g; 49% of calories

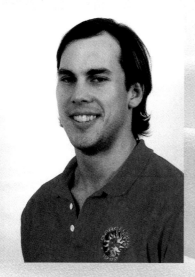

Danek Nowosielski
FENCING

Danek has been on the Canadian national team since 1985 and has competed in the 1988, 1992 and 1996 Olympics, the 1987, 1991 and 1995 Pan American Games (where he won one silver and three bronze medals), five World University Games (one silver medal), two Commonwealth championships (two gold medals) and nine world championships. He is a ten-time national champion.

Fluent in English, French and Polish, Danek is currently working on an M.Sc. in environmental geochemistry at McGill University in Montreal.

Danek's Pasta

Preparation time: 30 minutes

Quick and easy to prepare, this single-dish meal is low in fat and high in carbohydrates, and the mixture of vegetables contributes vitamins, minerals and fibre. Danek normally eats this for dinner before a competition or after a long training session.

14 oz.	tube-shaped pasta such as penne or ziti	400 g
2 Tbsp.	olive oil	25 mL
1 clove	garlic, pressed	1 clove
1	scallion, cut into thin diagonals	1
1 lb.	chicken breasts, boned, skinned and cut into thin strips	500 g
1 Tbsp.	mixed Italian herbs	15 mL
	salt	
	freshly ground black pepper	
½ each	large green, red and yellow peppers, cut into thin strips	½ each
3 Tbsp.	fresh lemon juice	40 mL
3 Tbsp.	water	40 mL
1 Tbsp.	thinly sliced scallion tops	15 mL
	grated Parmesan cheese	

Cook pasta to the *al dente* stage. Meanwhile, in a large skillet, heat oil, add garlic and scallion, and stir-fry for 1 minute. Add chicken, sprinkle with half the Italian seasoning, and add salt and pepper to taste. Stir-fry for 3 minutes. Add peppers, lemon juice, water, scallion tops and remaining Italian seasoning; stir. Cover, reduce heat, and simmer for 5 minutes. In a large bowl, mix pasta with chicken mixture. Serve with Parmesan cheese and freshly ground pepper. Serves 4.

Nutritional values per serving
(based on 4 servings):
calories: 323
fat: 11 g; 30% of calories
protein: 31 g; 39% of calories
carbohydrates: 25 g; 31% of calories

Shrimp Linguine

Preparation time: 30-40 minutes

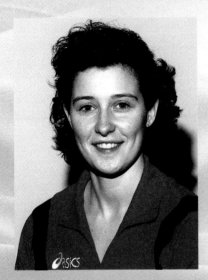

Lori Ann Mundt
V O L L E Y B A L L

"If I had to sum up my Olympic experience in one word," says Lori Ann, "it would be 'Wow!' To be a part of such a prestigious sporting event is quite an honour."

Lori Ann began playing volleyball at the age of 13. She has participated in the Atlanta Olympic Games, the Pan American Games in 1991 and 1995, the World Cup in 1991 and 1995, the World University Games in 1993 and 1995, the Canada Cup in 1993, 1994 and 1995 and Norceca in 1985, 1991 and 1993. She was coach of the Saskatchewan Midget Provincial B Team and an assistant coach for the University of Winnipeg women's volleyball team.

This is Lori Ann's favourite peak-performance dish because it tastes so good. She feels that anyone who loves shrimp will love this meal. It provides the carbo-loading you need either the day before or soon after a competition. She eats it anytime, though, not just for matches.

¼ cup	butter	50 mL
I	green pepper, chopped	I
½ cup	chopped onion	125 mL
14-oz. can	tomatoes, broken up	398 mL
1½ tsp.	garlic powder	7 mL
I tsp.	salt	5 mL
½ tsp.	oregano	2 mL
½ tsp.	basil	2 mL
¼ tsp.	pepper	1 mL
8 oz.	cocktail shrimp	250 g
7½-oz. can	tomato sauce	213 mL
2 tsp.	parsley flakes	10 mL
8 oz.	linguine	250 g
I Tbsp.	cooking oil	15 mL
2 tsp.	salt	10 mL
	Parmesan cheese (optional)	

Melt butter in saucepan. Add green pepper and onion, and sauté until soft. Add tomatoes, garlic powder, I tsp. salt, oregano, basil and pepper. Simmer, uncovered, for 10-20 minutes, or until juice is almost gone. Add shrimp, tomato sauce and parsley, and simmer for another 15 minutes. Meanwhile, cook linguine in boiling water with oil and 2 tsp. salt until tender but firm. Drain, and mix with sauce. Top with Parmesan cheese if desired. Serves 4.

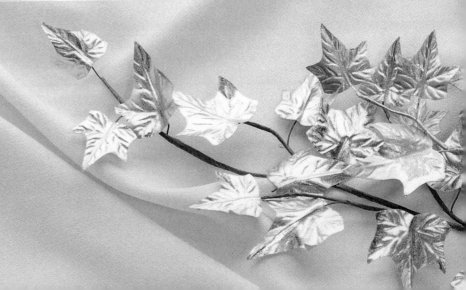

Nutritional values per serving
(based on 4 servings):
calories: 465
fat: 17 g; 34% of calories
protein: 22 g; 19% of calories
carbohydrates: 55 g; 47% of calories

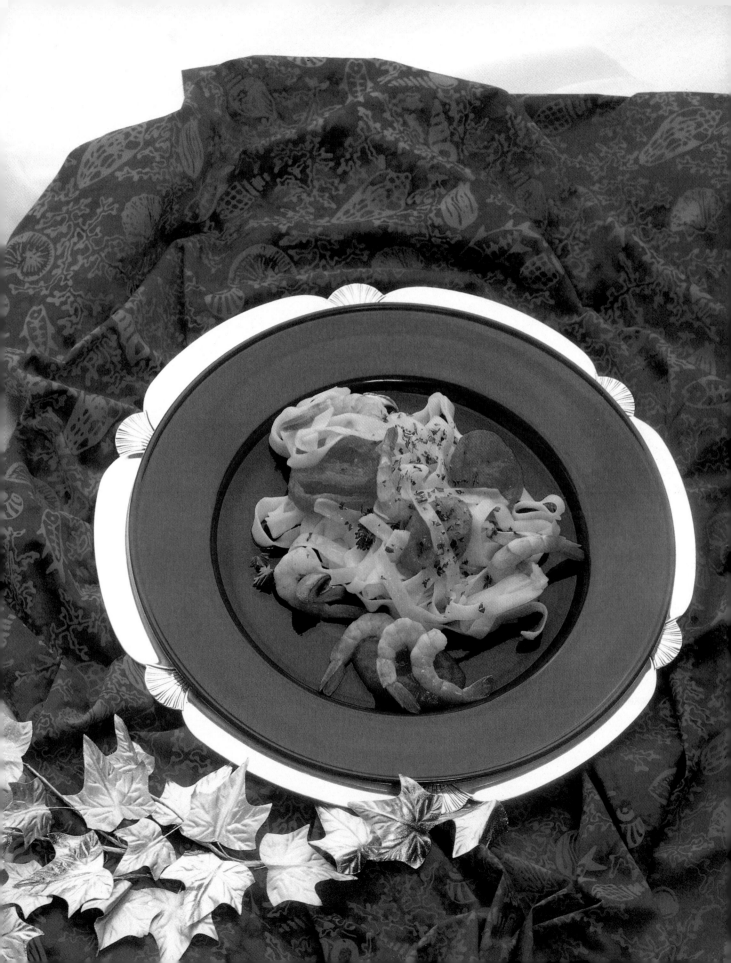

Annie's Seafood Surf-Prise

Preparation time: 30 minutes

"Seafood makes me dive like a fish," says Annie. "This is my favourite pre-event dish, and it makes me feel satisfied but not full. I normally eat this meal four hours before a competition. Right before competing, I eat fruit to calm my nerves and give me an energy boost."

14-oz. can	stewed tomatoes	398 mL
12	popcorn shrimp	12
1 cup	sliced mushrooms	250 mL
½	medium onion, chopped	½
12 oz.	linguine	340 g
½ tsp.	sugar	2 mL
½ tsp.	tarragon	2 mL
	salt and pepper	
	parsley	
	cayenne pepper	

Bring the stewed tomatoes to a slow boil, and simmer for 5 minutes, then reduce heat to medium-low. Add shrimp, mushrooms and onion, and simmer for 10 minutes. Meanwhile, cook the linguine in a large pot of boiling water until it is *al dente*. Add sugar and tarragon to sauce, then add salt, pepper, parsley and cayenne pepper to taste. Pour over the pasta, and serve. Serves 4.

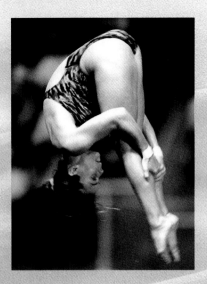

Annie Pelletier
DIVING

Annie has been a member of the Canadian national team since 1991 and had a tremendous 1996 Olympic Games, coming from behind to win a bronze medal in the three-metre dive competition. But this comes as no surprise: 1996 saw her take 1st place in the three-metre at both the Canadian national diving championships and the Pan American Games.

Annie was born in Montreal in 1973 and is a student at Collège André Grasset. Fluent in French, English and Spanish, she enjoys golf, writing, music and dance.

Nutritional values per serving
(based on 4 servings):
calories: 394
fat: 2 g; 5% of calories
protein: 21 g; 22% of calories
carbohydrates: 72 g; 73% of calories

Patrick's Salmon Dinner

Preparation time: 45 minutes

7½-oz. can	salmon	213 mL
2 tsp.	margarine	10 mL
¼ cup	chopped onion	50 mL
¼ cup	chopped celery	50 mL
¼ cup	chopped green pepper	50 mL
1 clove	garlic, minced	1 clove
3 cups	diced potatoes	750 mL
1 cup	diced carrots	250 mL
2 cups	chicken stock	500 mL
½ tsp.	pepper	2 mL
½ tsp.	dill seed	2 mL
1 cup	diced zucchini	250 mL
14-oz. can	evaporated milk	398 mL
10-oz. can	cream-style corn	284 mL
½ cup	chopped fresh parsley	125 mL

Drain and flake salmon, reserving liquid, and set both aside. In a large nonstick frying pan, melt margarine over medium heat. Add onion, celery, green pepper and garlic, and cook, stirring often, for 5 minutes, or until vegetables are tender. Add potatoes, carrot, chicken stock, pepper and dill seed. Bring to a full boil, then reduce heat, cover, and simmer for 20 minutes, or until vegetables are tender. Add zucchini, and simmer, covered, for 5 more minutes. Add salmon, reserved liquid, evaporated milk and corn. Cook over low heat just until heated through. Add parsley just before serving. Serves 4.

Patrick Newman
R O W I N G

Patrick has been rowing since 1980. In 1987, he placed 7th at the world championships in cox pair. At the 1988 Olympics, he came in 10th in the same event. At the world championships in 1992 and 1993, he placed 4th and 1st, respectively, in the lightweight 8+, and in 1995, he was 9th in the heavyweight 8+. In the 1996 Olympics, Patrick's heavyweight 8+ squad was 4th.

Nutritional values per serving
(based on 4 servings):
calories: 434
fat: 13 g; 27% of calories
protein: 21 g; 19% of calories
carbohydrates: 58 g; 53% of calories

The Vegetarian Challenge

Curried Lentils

Preparation time: 20 minutes

2½ cups	stock	625 mL
1 cup	lentils	250 mL
1	bay leaf	1
1 tsp.	salt	5 mL
3 Tbsp.	olive oil	40 mL
1	large onion, diced	1
3 cloves	garlic, crushed	3 cloves
2 tsp.	curry powder	10 mL
2 Tbsp.	lemon juice	25 mL

Bring stock to a boil, and add lentils, bay leaf and salt. Lower heat, cover and cook. Meanwhile, heat oil over medium heat in a frying pan, add onion, garlic and curry powder, and sauté until onion is translucent. Stir in lemon juice. Add onion mixture to cooked lentils. Serve over rice. Serves 2-4.

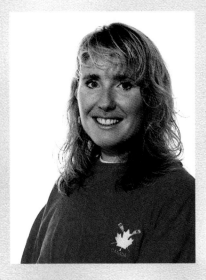

Theresa Luke
R O W I N G

Theresa started rowing at Simon Fraser University in 1991. At the 1996 Olympics in Atlanta, her team, the women's 8+, took the silver medal. She is interested in a healthy lifestyle centred around rowing her way to the 2000 Olympic Games in Sydney, Australia. She is also an avid horseback rider. Her plans for the future include setting up her own business.

Nutritional values per serving
(based on 4 servings; without rice):

calories: 318	
fat: 12 g; 34% of calories	
protein: 14 g; 18% of calories	
carbohydrates: 38 g; 48% of calories	

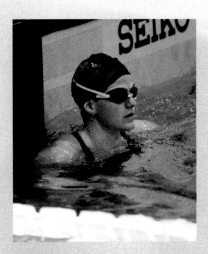

Nikki Dryden
S W I M M I N G

Nikki had been on the national swimming team for six years before the Atlanta Olympics, when she qualified in the 800-metre freestyle. She is a 16-time national champion and has held the Canadian short-course 400 freestyle record since 1993. Nikki is currently completing her studies in international relations and is hoping to pursue a diplomatic career. Both parents were athletes. Her mother was on the Canadian netball team and nearly made the 1968 Australian Olympic track and field team. Her father, also an Australian, represented Canada in international rugby competition.

Spanish Lentils

Preparation time: 40 minutes

This is Nikki's favourite recipe because it turns plain lentils into a wonderful high-energy dish. As a vegetarian, she eats it at least once a week during training. Brown rice or pasta, cooked appropriately, can be substituted for the lentils. (Jane Brody's recipe)

3 cups	water	750 mL
I cup	lentils	250 mL
I Tbsp.	olive oil	15 mL
4 cloves	garlic, chopped	4 cloves
½ cup	chopped green onions	125 mL
½ cup	chopped green peppers	125 mL
¼ tsp.	cumin	1 mL
I Tbsp.	chili powder	15 mL
8-oz. can	tomato paste	227 mL
I Tbsp.	red wine vinegar	15 mL

In a medium pot, combine water and lentils, and bring to a boil. Reduce heat to medium, cover, and simmer for 25 minutes. Meanwhile, heat oil in a saucepan, and sauté garlic, onions, green pepper, cumin and chili powder for 2 minutes. Stir in tomato paste and vinegar, and heat. When lentils are cooked, mix with the vegetables, and serve. Serves 4.

Nutritional values per serving
(based on 4 servings):
calories: 277
fat: 5 g; 16% of calories
protein: 16 g; 24% of calories
carbohydrates: 42 g; 60% of calories

Nikki's Performance Eating Tip:

Informed vegetarian eating can support a heavy training schedule, especially when one's diet is diverse.

Popeye's Pulse

Preparation time: 1½ hours

This is Jessica's favourite meal because it has a balance of carbohydrates and protein and is low in fat. Also, her vegetarian friends can join her. She eats it pre-event because it's light and doesn't add to the "butterflies" feeling she gets before a big race. The dish takes its name from two sources: Popeye's famous spinach, and "pulse," the word for edible seeds of legumes such as peas, beans or, in this case, lentils.

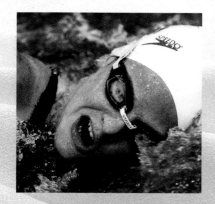

Jessica Amey
S W I M M I N G

1996 was Jessica's rookie year on the national swimming team. The Canadian record holder in the 100-metre butterfly, she began swimming competitively at age seven and now spends 20 hours a week training. She is at present surviving on Stanford University's cafeteria cuisine. By midterm, she says, "I would gladly trade my swim goggles for a home-cooked meal."

Jessica would love to become a chef. She knows that healthy eating contributes to fine performances, and she'd like to work with athletes to help them achieve personal bests with balanced, healthful menus.

8 cups	stock	2 L
2 cups	red lentils	500 mL
½ cup	brown rice	125 mL
2 cups	onions, finely chopped	500 mL
2 Tbsp.	olive oil	25 mL
3 cloves	garlic, minced	3 cloves
¼ tsp.	red pepper flakes	1 mL
½ tsp.	salt (or more as desired)	2 mL
2	bay leaves	2
¼ cup	fresh parsley, chopped	50 mL
pinch	rosemary	pinch
2 Tbsp.	lemon juice	25 mL
2 cups	chopped tomatoes	500 mL
2 cups	fresh spinach	500 mL

Pour the stock into a soup pot, add lentils and rice, and bring to a boil. Reduce heat and simmer, covered, for 1 hour. Meanwhile, in a nonstick frying pan, sauté onions in olive oil for 2 minutes. Add garlic, red pepper flakes, salt and bay leaves. Stir over medium heat until mixture is lightly browned. Add parsley, rosemary, lemon juice and tomatoes. When lentils are cooked, pour the onion-tomato mixture into the soup pot. Simmer for 15 minutes more. Just before serving, stir in fresh spinach. This meal goes well with a fresh salad and crusty rye bread. Serves 8.

Nutritional values per serving
(based on 8 servings):

calories: 321

fat: 7 g; 18% of calories

protein: 16 g; 20% of calories

carbohydrates: 50 g; 62% of calories

Carey Nelson's Blazin' Beans

Preparation time: 45 minutes

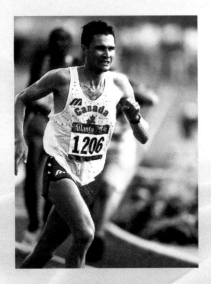

Carey Nelson
R U N N I N G

Carey has been a member of more than 20 Canadian national teams, including the 1988 Olympic team 5,000-metre, the 1996 Olympic team marathon and the 1994 Commonwealth Games marathon. His personal best in the marathon is 2:12:00, or 5:03 minutes per mile, for 26-plus miles.

He completed an M.B.A. at the University of British Columbia in 1991 and is currently taking courses from the Canadian Securities Institute. He owns a software company.

Carey says, "We (my wife Kate and I) cook Blazin' Beans once a week. I am not a vegetarian, but I do not like to eat meat every day, so we make Blazin' Beans. It is a good source of protein and easy to make. I would not recommend eating it the night before a race."

I	medium onion, coarsely chopped	I
I Tbsp.	sesame oil	15 mL
6 cloves	garlic, whole	6 cloves
2	hot red chilies, crushed	2
10-oz. can	black beans	284 mL
14-oz. can	*light* coconut milk	398 mL
I	medium zucchini, sliced	I
2 Tbsp.	soy sauce	25 mL
	salt and pepper	

Sauté onion over medium heat in sesame oil. Stir in garlic and chilies. Add black beans, coconut milk, zucchini and soy sauce. Simmer for 30 minutes, stirring frequently. Add salt and pepper to taste. Pour over a bed of brown rice. Serves 4.

Nutritional values per serving
(based on 4 servings):
calories: 239
fat: 9 g; 34% of calories
protein: 9 g; 15% of calories
carbohydrates: 31 g; 51% of calories

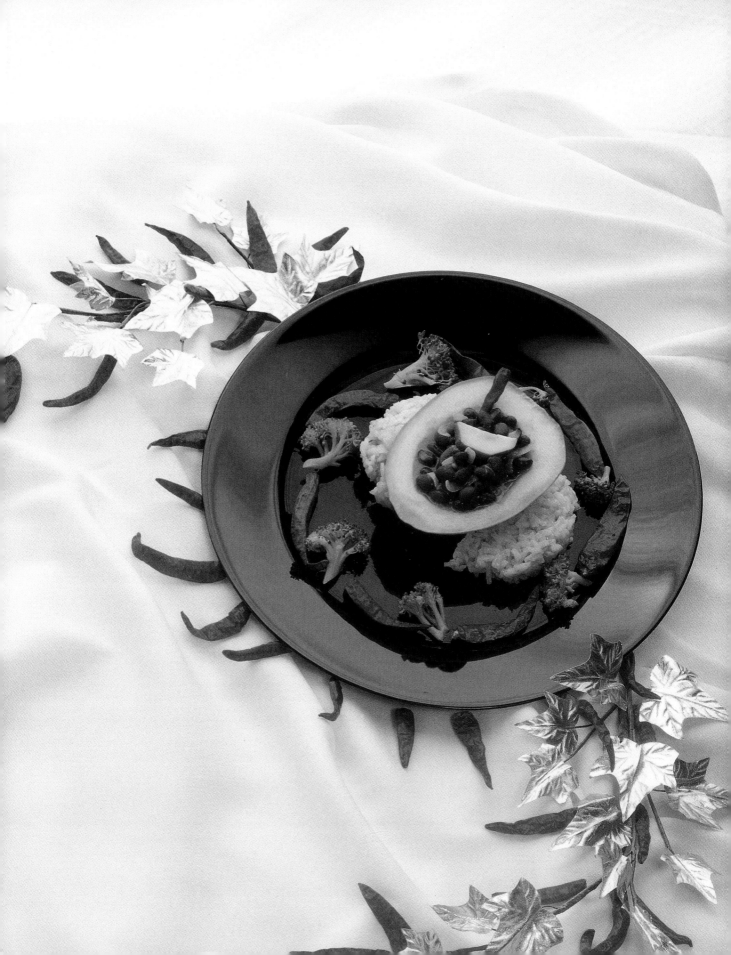

Frappé-la-Rue Couscous

Preparation time: 15 minutes

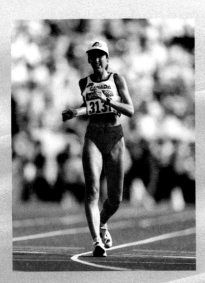

Tina Poitras
R A C E W A L K I N G

Tina has competed in the 10-km walk in two Olympic Games (1992 and 1996). Her career highlights include victories at the Hildesheim European Grand Prix (Germany) and the Hildesheim International Circuit (Japan, 1994). She is the 1995 and 1996 Canadian champion.

This is Tina's favourite peak-performance recipe because it is quick and easy to make and a winner every time with family and friends. She always eats it 12 to 14 hours before a competition.

2 cups	vegetable stock	500 mL
2 cups	couscous	500 mL
3 Tbsp.	olive oil	40 mL
2 cups	snow peas	500 mL
I stalk	celery, chopped	I stalk
I cup	broccoli florets	250 mL
I	red bell pepper, chopped	I
I	zucchini, sliced	I
2	medium onions, chopped	2
I Tbsp.	tamari sauce	15 mL
pinch	salt	pinch
pinch	cayenne pepper	pinch

Bring stock to a boil, then remove pot from the heat. Stir in couscous, cover pot, and let stand for 5 minutes. Place oil in frying pan over medium heat. Add vegetables, sauté for I minute, and combine with couscous. Add tamari sauce, salt and cayenne pepper. Serve hot or cold. Serves 6.

Nutritional values per serving
(based on 6 servings):

calories: 392	
fat: 8 g; 19% of calories	
protein: 12 g; 13% of calories	
carbohydrates: 67 g; 68% of calories	

Tina's Performance Eating Tip:

To optimize the energy in a carbohydrate meal, eat it 12 to 14 hours before your competition.

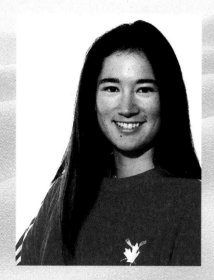

Tosha Tsang
R O W I N G

Like many rowers, Tosha was introduced to the sport at university. She rowed for four years with the McGill University team and, in 1992, began rowing full-time and trying out for the national rowing team. In 1995, she made the squad of the Women's 8+. In 1996, they won a silver medal at the Games in Atlanta to go with another silver earlier that year at the Rotsee Regatta in Lucerne, Switzerland.

Nutritional values per serving
(based on 6 servings):
calories: 552
fat: 21 g; 34% of calories
protein: 19 g; 14% of calories
carbohydrates: 72 g; 52% of calories

Chameleon Couscous

Preparation time: 1½–2½ hours

This is Tosha's favourite recipe because it is so versatile and healthful. The sauce aside, it can be made very quickly, and the ingredients can be changed according to taste.

1½ cups	water	375 mL
1½ cups	couscous	375 mL
1 Tbsp.	olive oil	15 mL
2 cloves	garlic, crushed	2 cloves
½ cup	mushrooms	125 mL
1 each	green, red and yellow bell peppers, cubed	1 each
1	medium zucchini, sliced	1
4 Tbsp.	Peanut-Ginger Sauce (see below)	50 mL

Bring water to a boil, add couscous, stir, and remove from heat. Cover and set aside for 5 minutes. Heat oil in a wok or frying pan over medium-high heat. Add garlic, then quickly add vegetables, and stir-fry for 30 seconds. Add Peanut-Ginger Sauce, and mix for 10 seconds. Remove from heat. Fluff couscous with a fork, and dish onto plates. Pour vegetables over the top. Serve immediately. Serves 6.

Peanut-Ginger Sauce (William Mohns' recipe):

¾ cup	natural peanut butter (crunchy)	150 mL
½ cup	honey	125 mL
3 cloves	garlic, chopped	3 cloves
½ tsp.	grated ginger	2 mL
⅓ cup	soy sauce	75 mL
	freshly ground pepper	
1 cup	medium-firm tofu, cubed	250 mL
½ cup	mushrooms	125 mL

Melt peanut butter and honey together. Add garlic, ginger and soy sauce and pepper to taste. Simmer over low heat for 20 minutes. Remove from heat, and allow to cool until lukewarm. Pour over tofu, and marinate for 45 minutes to 2 hours. After tofu has marinated, sauté mushrooms in a nonstick frying pan. Add tofu and marinade, and reheat thoroughly.

Tosha's Performance Eating Tip:

To get the most out of what you eat, select foods that are as close to their natural state as possible. Also, eat a variety of foods, especially fruits and vegetables.

Super Veggie Skillet Dinner

Preparation time: 40 minutes

Alison finds this to be her favourite peak-performance dish, providing vegetables, carbohydrates and protein without meat. She usually eats it for lunch or dinner after a hard workout.

5	large baking potatoes, cubed	5
1 bunch	broccoli, finely chopped	1 bunch
1 Tbsp.	oil	15 mL
1 each	red and yellow peppers, chopped	1 each
1	onion, chopped	1
2 cloves	garlic, minced	2 cloves
8 oz.	cheddar cheese, grated	250 g

Boil potatoes for 8 minutes or until almost tender. Add broccoli, and cook for 4-5 minutes. Drain. Heat oil in large, deep frying pan. Add potatoes, broccoli and all remaining ingredients except cheese. Cook until potatoes are golden and other vegetables are heated through. Add half of the grated cheese, and heat, stirring, until melted. Sprinkle top with remaining cheese. Cover pan to melt cheese for 3-4 minutes. Serves 6.

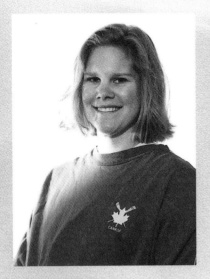

Alison Korn
R O W I N G

An all-round athlete who has competed at the varsity level in both basketball and ice hockey, Alison began rowing in 1992 at McGill University. 1996 was her first year on the national team, which earned silver at the Olympic Games. She has competed in both the women's 8+ and the women's 4+. She is currently training for the 2000 Olympic Games.

Alison completed her B.A. in political science (honours) at McGill University in 1993 and is currently completing a master's degree in journalism at Carleton University.

Nutritional values per serving
(based on 6 servings):
calories: 410
fat: 15 g; 34% of calories
protein: 16 g; 16% of calories
carbohydrates: 52 g; 50% of calories

Alison's Performance Eating Tip:

Eat a good, substantial breakfast, then pack a lunch so that you won't be tempted to buy junk food.

Finish-Fast Feta Pasta

Preparation time: 15 minutes

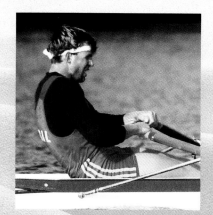

This is Todd's favourite recipe because it is nutritious and fast and simple to prepare. He normally eats it for dinner a couple of nights before an event.

30 oz.	penne pasta	900 g
1 tsp.	olive oil	5 mL
8	tomatoes, cut in wedges	8
¼ cup	fresh basil	50 mL
½ cup	fresh parsley	125 mL
10 oz.	feta cheese	300 g
¼ cup	pitted black olives	50 mL
	freshly ground black pepper	

Cook pasta until it is *al dente*. Meanwhile, heat oil in a large skillet. Add tomatoes, and cook at medium-high heat for 4 minutes. Strain pasta, and mix with tomatoes, basil and parsley. Crumble feta on top, garnish with olives, and season with black pepper to taste. Serves 4-6.

Todd Hallett
R O W I N G

Todd was first introduced to the sport of rowing as a spectator at a Canada Day regatta in Dartmouth, Nova Scotia. Shortly thereafter, he took a friend up on an offer to give it a try. Hallett was a natural and went on to win gold in both the single and double at the 1988 junior national championships, as well as Junior Sculler of the Year. He has been on the national team since 1991 and has been national champion on several occasions. At both the 1992 and 1996 Olympic Games, Todd placed 7th in the men's double. Also in 1996, he placed 4th in both the Lucerne and Duisburg international regattas.

Nutritional values per serving
(based on 6 servings):
calories: 319
fat: 12 g; 35% of calories
protein: 11 g; 14% of calories
carbohydrates: 41 g; 51% of calories

Vegetarian Lasagna

Preparation time: 1½ hours

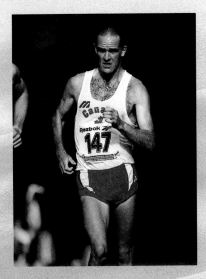

Tim Berrett
R A C E W A L K I N G

Tim is number one in Canada's 50-km racewalk. He is also a high achiever academically. While walking his way to the 1995 and 1996 Canadian championship, he was putting the finishing touches on his Ph.D. at the University of Alberta.

Tim believes in doing as well in school as in sports and takes time to visit schools to give students a firsthand account of the kind of commitment it takes to reach the top in both sports and education.

This is Tim's favourite peak-performance recipe because it is tasty and provides all the essential nutrients and carbohydrates. He normally eats it prior to a race or post-workout for replenishment.

8 oz.	lasagna noodles	250 g
2 tsp.	oil	10 mL
2 cloves	garlic, chopped	2 cloves
½ lb.	mushrooms, sliced	250 g
1	green pepper, chopped	1
2	onions, chopped	2
28-oz. can	tomatoes	796 mL
14-oz. can	tomato sauce	398 mL
2	carrots, shredded	2
1 tsp.	oregano	5 mL
¼ cup	chopped parsley	50 mL
1 tsp.	basil	5 mL
1 tsp.	crushed chilies	5 mL
1 lb.	ricotta cheese	500 g
10 oz.	spinach, chopped	300 g
2	eggs	2
1 cup	Parmesan cheese	250 mL
1 cup	grated mozzarella cheese	250 mL

Cook noodles in boiling water. Drain and set aside. Heat oil in frying pan, add garlic, mushrooms, green pepper and onions, and cook for 5 minutes. Add tomatoes, tomato sauce, carrots and seasonings. Cook for 30 minutes. In a bowl, combine ricotta, spinach, eggs and half the Parmesan cheese. Spread a thin layer of sauce in the bottom of a lasagna pan, then layer in the other ingredients: half of each of the noodles, ricotta mixture, sauce and mozzarella. Repeat the layers, and top with the remaining Parmesan cheese. Bake at 350°F (180°C) for 30 minutes. Cover and cook for 20 minutes more. Let stand for a few minutes before serving. Serves 8.

Nutritional values per serving
(based on 8 servings):
calories: 326
fat: 17 g; 48% of calories
protein: 20 g; 25% of calories
carbohydrates: 22 g; 27% of calories

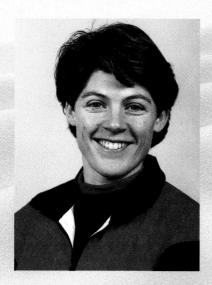

Juanita Clayton
S O F T B A L L

Juanita's athletic career is full of triumphs. Her team placed 5th in the 1996 Olympics, 4th in the 1994 world championships in St. John's, Newfoundland, and 2nd and 4th, respectively, in the 1991 and 1995 Pan American Games. In 1995 and 1996, her team won the Canadian championship, and she was named All-Star Catcher in 1995 and most valuable player of the playoff round in 1996.

Lasagna

Preparation time: 1½ hours

This is Juanita's favourite recipe because it is delicious, high in carbohydrates and full of vitamins and minerals. She normally eats it the night before a major event.

8 oz.	lasagna noodles	250 g
2 cups	sliced, unpeeled zucchini	500 mL
½ cup	sliced mushrooms	125 mL
	any other vegetables desired	
2 cups	tomato sauce	500 mL
1½ cups	part-skim ricotta cheese	375 mL
½ cup	shredded part-skim mozzarella cheese	125 mL
2 Tbsp.	Parmesan cheese	25 mL

Preheat oven to 400°F (200°C). Cook lasagna noodles until chewy (about 10 minutes); drain and cool. Place a third of noodles, slightly overlapping, in bottom of baking dish. Layer remaining ingredients as follows: zucchini, mushrooms and any other vegetables desired, 1½ cups tomato sauce, a third of the noodles, ricotta cheese, mozzarella cheese, remaining noodles, remaining tomato sauce and Parmesan cheese. Cover with aluminum foil, and bake for 30 minutes; uncover and bake for another 30 minutes. Serves 8.

Nutritional values per serving	
(based on 8 servings):	
calories: 222	
fat: 6 g; 25% of calories	
protein: 13 g; 23% of calories	
carbohydrates: 29 g; 52% of calories	

Juanita's Performance Eating Tip:

Healthy eating doesn't mean giving up taste. Healthy eating combined with a moderate exercise plan will lift your spirits and lengthen your life.

Spinach Lasagna

Preparation time: 1 hour

After a good day on the slopes, this warm and tasty dish is sure to hit the spot.

1 lb.	ricotta cheese	500 g
10-oz pkg.	frozen spinach (thawed)	284 mL
2	medium eggs	2
8 oz.	sliced mozzarella cheese	250 g
8 oz.	lasagna	250 g
28-oz. tin	crushed tomatoes	796 mL
	oregano, basil, garlic powder	
	and salt and pepper to taste	

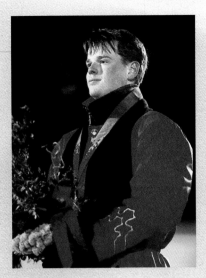

Jean-Luc Brassard
FREESTYLE SKIING

Jean-Luc began skiing at the age of seven and, by the time he was 18, had won his first World Cup. He boasts an impressive list of victories, including 40 World Cup medals, three overall crowns and world titles in 1993 and 1997. Three times, Jean-Luc has been awarded the John Semmelink Trophy, which is presented each year to the skier who best represents Canada in international competition through his or her sports- manship, good conduct and fine performance.

Cook pasta according to package directions, cool and drain. In a large bowl, combine the spinach, ricotta cheese and eggs. In a separate bowl combine tomatoes and seasonings. Place a little sauce on the bottom of a baking pan to prevent the noodles from sticking. Next add a layer of noodles, half the ricotta mixture and half the mozzarella. Repeat. Bake in a preheated oven for 45 minutes at 350°F (180°C). Let rest for 5 minutes before cutting. Serves 8.

Nutritional values per serving
(based on 8 servings):
calories: 316
fat: 13 g; 37% of calories
protein: 19 g; 24% of calories
carbohydrates: 30 g; 39% of calories

Spin-the-Tires Fusilli

Preparation time: 20-30 minutes

This is Alison's favourite peak-performance recipe because it is very tasty and easy to prepare — especially when travelling, as it doesn't require much in the way of kitchen accessories. She will eat it prior to or even after an event. It tastes good hot or cold.

1 lb.	fusilli	500 g
6-8	mushrooms, chopped	6-8
1 Tbsp.	olive oil	15 mL
6	Roma tomatoes, chopped	6
2 cloves	garlic, crushed	2 cloves
½ cup	crumbled feta cheese	125 mL
½ cup	fresh parsley	125 mL
2 Tbsp.	fresh basil, chopped	25 mL
½ cup	grated fresh Parmesan cheese, freshly ground pepper	125 mL

Cook pasta, drain, and return to warm pot. In a nonstick skillet, sauté mushrooms in olive oil over medium heat. Add tomatoes, and cook, stirring, for 2 minutes. Add garlic, and cook until tomatoes are heated through. Add vegetables to pasta along with feta, parsley, basil and Parmesan. Toss lightly. Add freshly ground pepper to taste, and serve. Serves 4.

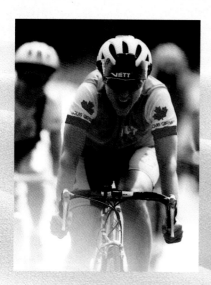

Alison Sydor
C Y C L I N G

Going into Atlanta, Alison was ranked number one in the world in women's mountain biking, and she didn't disappoint, winning a silver medal in XC mountain biking. She has won 12 Canadian national championship titles and many other regional and international titles. Alison has a degree in biochemistry from the University of Victoria.

Nutritional values per serving
(based on 4 servings):
calories: 584
fat: 12 g; 19% of calories
protein: 24 g; 16% of calories
carbohydrates: 94 g; 65% of calories

Alison's Performance Eating Tip:

To maintain your edge all day long, eat several modest servings of high-quality whole foods throughout the day.

Tagliatelle Verdi

Preparation time: 15 minutes

Cynthia enjoys this meal because it is quick, savoury and easy to digest. It is also a way of carbo-loading for vegetarians and non-vegetarians alike. She normally eats this 4 to 5 hours before a game.

3 oz.	tagliatelle verdi	85 g
¼ cup	sun-dried tomatoes	125 mL
¼ cup	olive oil	125 mL
	goat cheese, cream cheese	
	or Parmesan cheese	

Cook noodles for 3-5 minutes in boiling water. Cut up tomatoes while waiting for the pasta to cook. Drain pasta, and place in a bowl. Add olive oil, tomatoes and cheese to taste. Serves 1-2.

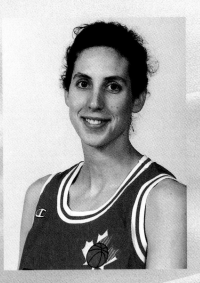

Cynthia Johnston
BASKETBALL

Cynthia has been in the Canadian Women's National Basketball Program since she was 16 years old. After several tries, the women's team qualified for the 1996 Olympics in Atlanta. Cynthia played four years of professional basketball in Belgium.

She grew up in Rothesay, New Brunswick, and studied art history and history at Bishop's University. She now lives (and still plays) in Switzerland. She has been a vegetarian for five years.

Nutritional values per serving
(based on 2 servings):
calories: 415
fat: 31 g; 66% of calories
protein: 7 g; 7% of calories
carbohydrates: 27 g; 27% of calories

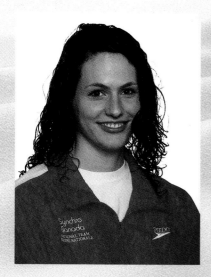

Karen Clark
SYNCHRONIZED SWIMMING

When she was 12 years old, Karen was the youngest swimmer ever to win an individual national title in her sport, and she went on to win three more. She won the silver medal at the 1996 Olympics and is now ranked 2nd in the world. She attends the University of Calgary as a two-time recipient of the Petro-Canada Olympic Torch Scholarship and participates in the Adopt-An-Athlete Program.

Delicious Pizza

Preparation time: 30 minutes

This is Karen's favourite peak-performance recipe because it's full of vegetables and tastes good.

14-oz. can	low-fat tomato sauce	398 mL
½ clove	garlic, crushed	½ clove
	basil and oregano	
10-inch	pizza crust	25 cm
8	mushrooms, chopped	8
½	red pepper, chopped	½
½	green pepper, chopped	½
1	onion, chopped	1
	grated Parmesan or low-fat cheddar cheese	

Place tomato sauce in a small bowl. Add garlic, then basil and oregano to taste. Spread sauce over crust, and arrange vegetables on top. Sprinkle with Parmesan or low-fat cheddar. Cook in 325°F (160°C) oven for 20 minutes. Serves 2.

Nutritional values per serving
(based on 2 servings):
calories: 470
fat: 6 g; 11% of calories
protein: 18 g; 15% of calories
carbohydrates: 87 g; 74% of calories

Karen's Performance Eating Tip:

Eat what you love, but be mindful of eating too much fat.

Broccoli and Tofu Quiche

Preparation time: 45 minutes

Myriam loves this recipe because it is easy to prepare and is a complete meal in one dish. For variety, try adding mushrooms or substituting asparagus for the broccoli.

9-inch	pie shell, uncooked	23 cm
2 cups	broccoli florets, cooked, drained and cooled	500 mL
4 oz.	firm tofu, drained and diced	125 g
I cup	grated Swiss cheese	250 mL
4	medium eggs	4
I cup	milk	250 mL
I clove	garlic, crushed	I clove
I tsp.	chopped coriander leaves (cilantro)	5 mL

Precook pie shell in 350°F (180°C) oven for 5 minutes or until the pastry has formed a slight skin. Remove from oven, and cool for I minute. Arrange broccoli, tofu and cheese in pie shell. In a bowl, whisk eggs, then add milk, garlic and coriander. Pour over ingredients in pie shell. Bake in a preheated 350°F (180°C) oven for 25 minutes. Remove from oven, and let rest before slicing. Serves 6.

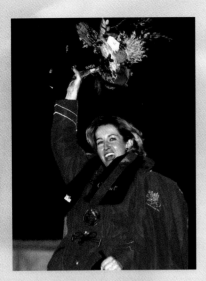

Myriam Bédard
BIATHLON

Myriam began competing at the age of 16, and has been a national team member since 1987. Born just outside of Quebec City, she has participated in a variety of sports during her 29 years, including: figure skating, basketball, swimming, windsurfing, and ballet, to name just a few. Besides having several Olympic medals to her credit, she was also Biathlon Canada's athlete of the year for four years in a row (1991 - 1994). Her husband (Jean) and her daughter (Maude) traditionally accompany her to every competition.

Nutritional values per serving
(based on 6 servings):
calories: 328
fat: 21 g; 57% of calories
protein: 15 g; 19% of calories
carbohydrates: 20 g; 24% of calories

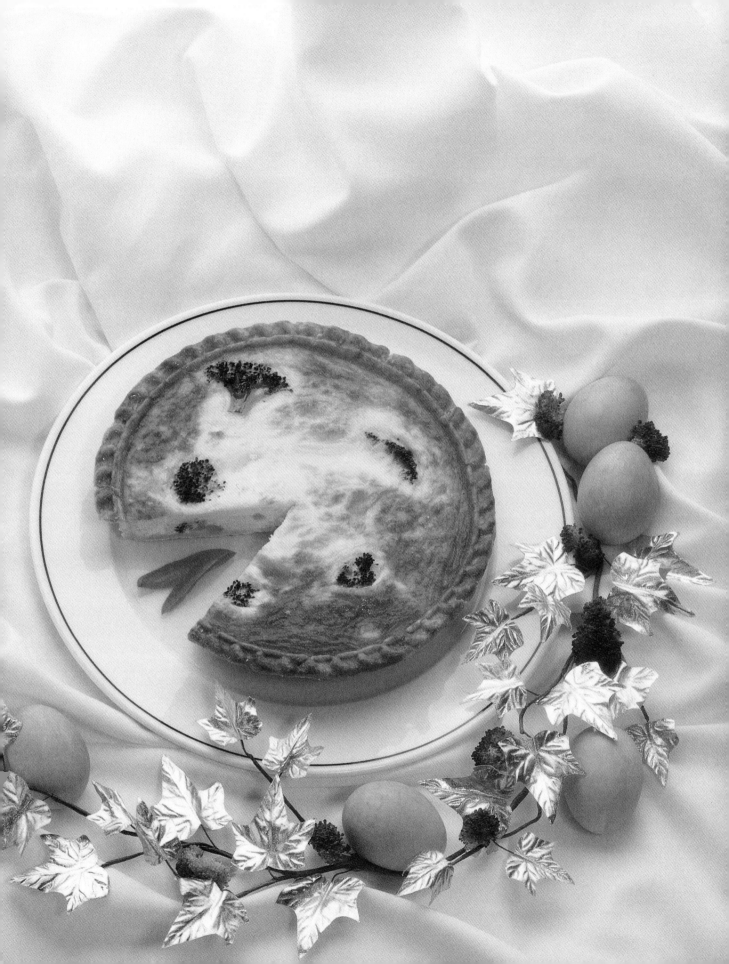

Pizza Bread

Preparation time: 45 minutes

This is Riley's favourite recipe because it is easy to make, tastes good and is high in carbohydrates. She normally eats it for dinner the day before a race.

Crust:

2½ cups	flour	625 mL
I Tbsp.	vegetable oil	15 mL
I Tbsp.	fast-rising yeast	15 mL
I Tbsp.	salt	15 mL
I cup	warm water	250 mL

Topping:

¼ tsp.	salt	I mL
¼ tsp.	thyme	I mL
¼ tsp.	oregano	I mL
¼ tsp.	garlic powder	I mL
pinch	pepper	pinch
⅓ cup	golden Italian dressing	75 mL
½ cup	Parmesan cheese	125 mL
½ cup	grated mozzarella cheese	125 mL

Mix all ingredients for crust in a large bowl. Cover, and let rise for 20 minutes. Spread over greased pizza pan. Combine seasonings in a small bowl. Brush Italian dressing over dough, sprinkle seasonings on top, then Parmesan and mozzarella cheese. Cook in 450°F (230°C) oven for 10-15 minutes. Serves 6.

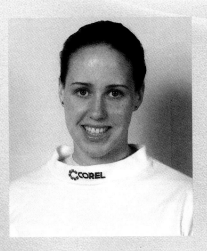

Riley Mants
S W I M M I N G

1996 was a big year for Riley. She competed in the 200-metre breaststroke for Canada at the Atlanta Games, was the 200-metre U.S. winter national champion (the first Canadian swimmer in 20 years to win a U.S. national title) and was honoured with three awards: the Victor Davis Memorial Scholarship Award, Manitoba's Youth Athlete of the Year and Manitoba's Swimmer of the Year. In 1995, Riley was a member of the Pan-Pacific Team in Atlanta, the Canadian national champion in 200-metre breaststroke in Winnipeg and a member of the 1994/95 Canadian junior national team.

Nutritional values per serving
(based on 6 servings):
calories: 336
fat: 14 g; 37% of calories
protein: 11 g; 13% of calories
carbohydrates: 42 g; 50% of calories

Crowd Pleasers

Chilled Gazpacho

Preparation time: 3 hours

6	tomatoes, peeled and seeded	6
I	medium cucumber, peeled and seeded	I
I	green pepper, chopped	I
I	small onion, diced	I
½ cup	chopped celery	125 mL
I clove	garlic, crushed	I clove
I tsp.	salt	5 mL
2 Tbsp.	basil	25 mL
½ tsp.	paprika	2 mL
½ cup	tomato juice	125 mL
⅓ cup	extra-virgin olive oil	75 mL
3 Tbsp.	lemon juice	40 mL
	parsley	
	croutons (see recipe below)	

In a bowl, combine vegetables with garlic, salt, basil and paprika. In 4 batches, blend mixture in a food processor to a thick, chunky consistency. Add tomato juice, olive oil and lemon juice to the final batch before processing. Mix all batches together, and chill for 2-3 hours. Garnish with parsley and croutons (recipe below), and serve. Serves 4.

Croutons:

I clove	garlic, chopped	I clove
½ tsp.	extra-virgin olive oil	2 mL
5 slices	bread, cubed	5 slices

Sauté garlic in olive oil over medium heat. Add bread cubes, and sauté until lightly browned and crisp.

Peeling a Tomato: A Non-Olympic Moment

There are two ways to peel a tomato—the hard way and the easy way. Here's the easy way: Cut an X just through the skin at the bottom end of the tomato. Place the tomato on the end of a long-handled fork, and immerse it in boiling water for 30 seconds. Remove from water, and dip it in cold water for a couple of minutes. Peel away the skin, starting at the X. The hard way? You don't really want to know.

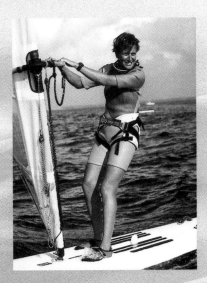

Caroll-Ann Alie
Y A C H T I N G

A member of Canada's sailing team since 1983, Caroll-Ann is a two-time Olympian (1992 and 1996) and a three-time world windsurfing champion (1984, 1985 and 1988). She was also the Canadian Yachting Association's Female Athlete of the Year for a remarkable eight years running, from 1988 to 1995. In 1993, she was inducted into the Canadian Amateur Sports Hall of Fame. In 1996, Caroll-Ann won gold at the Canadian Olympic Trials in Florida and took bronze medals in three separate international regattas. She is a registered dietitian.

Nutritional values per serving
(based on 4 servings; includes croutons):
calories: 353
fat: 20 g; 52% of calories
protein: 6 g; 7% of calories
carbohydrates: 36 g; 41% of calories

Oriental Soup

Preparation time: 20 minutes

This is my favourite recipe....I just LOVE Asian noodles! I eat this at least twice a week because it is easy, fast, nutritious, and low in fat.

3 cups	water	750 mL
½ inch	ginger root, thinly sliced	I cm
I tsp.	garlic, chopped	5 mL
6	mushrooms, chopped	6
½ cup	corn (canned or frozen)	125 mL
½ cup	bok choy (Chinese cabbage), shredded	125 mL
pinch	saffron	pinch
6 Tbsp.	powdered chicken soup stock	75 mL
	oregano, salt and pepper to taste	
I pkg.	oriental noodles, any flavour	I pkg.
½ cup	shrimp or chicken	125 mL
½ cup	bean sprouts	125 mL
6	mint leaves	6

Into water, place all ingredients except last four. Bring to a boil, then simmer for 5 minutes. Add meat and noodles, and cook for an additional 3-5 minutes. Finally, add the bean sprouts and mint leaves. Serve in a large Chinese soup bowl.

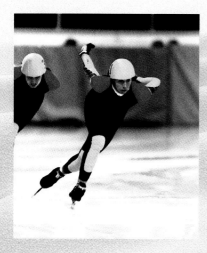

Nathalie Lambert
S P E E D
S K A T I N G

Nathalie, a 35 year old native of Montreal, Québec, holds both Canadian and World records in the 1500m and 1000m respectively. After a two year break from skating, during which she concentrated on motivational speaking engagements, Nathalie is back in the world of competition. Unfortunately, she was unable to compete in the Nagano Games because of a broken ankle.

Nathalie continues to encourage amateur athletes by managing an annual golf tournament to raise funds for speed skaters.

Nutritional values per serving
(based on 4 servings):

calories: 364

fat: 15 g; 36% of calories

protein: 12 g; 14% of calories

carbohydrates: 45 g; 50% of calories

Zucchini Soup

Preparation time: 20 minutes

This is Claire's favourite peak-performance dish because it is so easy to make that it is always available. It's good hot or cold.

1	onion, chopped	1
2 tsp.	butter	10 mL
3	medium zucchini, unpeeled, thickly sliced	3
1 cup	stock	250 mL
	cumin	
	curry powder	
	salt and pepper	
	additional stock or milk	
	chopped chives	

Sauté onion in butter until golden. Add zucchini and stock. Bring to a boil, and simmer until zucchini is very soft. Blend in food processor or with a hand mixer until smooth. Add seasonings to taste and more stock (or milk) until desired consistency is reached. Sprinkle with chives, and serve hot or cold. Serves 2.

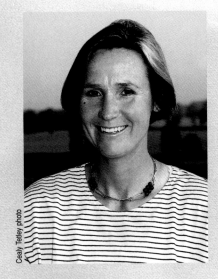

Cealy Telley photo

Claire Smith
E Q U E S T R I A N

Claire represented Canada in the equestrian three-day event at the 1996 Olympics. In 1995, she placed 6th and was top Canadian at the Fairhill, Maryland, three-day event. In 1994, she received the Cities of Ottawa, Nepean and Gloucester Sports Award and was the only three-day-event rider to qualify two horses at the World Equestrian Games. In 1993, Claire ranked 5th in North America and 9th in world newcomers. In 1992, she won the Furtive Trophy for highest-placed foreign rider at Fairhill.

Nutritional values per serving
(based on 2 servings):
calories: 143
fat: 5 g; 34% of calories
protein: 7 g; 19% of calories
carbohydrates: 17 g; 47% of calories

Orzo Soup

Preparation time: 1¼ hours

"You'll wish your pot was bigger," says Corrina. This is her favourite recipe because it makes a big batch to refrigerate or freeze. She just heats it up in the microwave for a quick, healthful lunch.

½ cup	butter	125 mL
2	medium onions, finely chopped	2
1	medium green pepper, finely chopped	1
2	carrots, finely chopped	2
2	celery stalks, chopped	2
1 clove	garlic, finely chopped	1 clove
19-oz. can	tomatoes	540 mL
10 cups	water or tomato juice	2.5 L
½ cup	chicken stock	125 mL
1 tsp.	garlic salt	5 mL
½ tsp.	oregano	2 mL
½ tsp.	black pepper	2 mL
pinch	ground cloves	pinch
1 cup	orzo noodles	250 mL
3-4 Tbsp.	Worcestershire sauce	40-50 mL
½ tsp.	mint	2 mL
	salt	

Melt butter in a saucepan large enough for finished soup. Add onions, green pepper, carrots, celery and garlic. Cook over medium heat, covered, until soft — at least 30 minutes — stirring occasionally. Add tomatoes, and cook for another 5 minutes. Add water or tomato juice, chicken stock, garlic salt, oregano, pepper and cloves. Bring to a boil, then add noodles. Simmer for 30 minutes, then add Worcestershire sauce, mint and salt to taste. Serves 12.

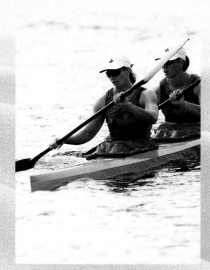

Corrina Kennedy
CANOEING

Corrina started paddling in the summer of 1987, and she made the national team in 1990. Her first International meet was the 1991 Pan American Games in Cuba, where she won the K-1 and K-2 500-metre and placed 2nd in the K-4 500-metre. In 1995, her team placed 1st in the K-2 and K-4 200-metre at the world championships, and the women's kayak team was named the best female Canadian team of the year at the Canadian Sport Awards. In 1996, she raced the K-2 and K-4 500-metre at the Olympic games and placed 5th in both events.

Corrina's Performance Eating Tip:

Snack on arrowroot cookies and apples so that you won't be tempted to buy potato chips.

Nutritional values per serving
(based on 12 servings; with V-8 juice):
calories: 208
fat: 9 g; 37% of calories
protein: 5 g; 9% of calories
carbohydrates: 28 g; 54% of calories

Virtuous Turkey Soup With Tomato and Fresh Basil

Preparation time: 30 minutes

This is Janice's favourite peak-performance dish because it is tasty and nutritious — perfect post-event or after a long workout. She serves it with warm rolls and salad to make it a complete meal.

I Tbsp.	olive oil	I5 mL
I lb.	ground turkey	500 g
I	onion, finely chopped	I
2 cloves	garlic, finely chopped	2 cloves
2 cups	coarsely chopped cabbage	500 mL
6 cups	chicken stock	I.5 L
28-oz. can	stewed tomatoes	796 mL
½ cup	orzo noodles	I25 mL
2 Tbsp.	fresh basil, chopped	25 mL
	salt and pepper	
	grated Parmesan cheese	

In a large saucepan, heat oil over medium heat. Add turkey, and sauté for 3-4 minutes or until no longer pink. Using a slotted spoon, remove turkey from pan. Add onion and garlic to pan, and sauté for 2 minutes. Add cabbage; sauté I minute. Stir in stock and tomatoes, and bring to a boil. Add noodles, and boil gently for I5 minutes or until tender, stirring occasionally. Add turkey and basil, heat through, and add salt and pepper to taste. Serve with a sprinkling of Parmesan cheese on top. Serves 8.

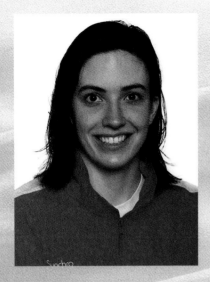

Janice Bremner
SYNCHRONIZED SWIMMING

A competitive synchronized swimmer since the age of nine, Janice has been a member of the Canadian national team since 1990 and realized a lifelong dream when she competed at the 1996 Olympic Games. In 1994, her team took a 2nd in the world championships, and in 1995, they placed 1st in the Canadian championships and 2nd in the World Cup. Janice was the recipient of a Petro-Canada Olympic Torch Scholarship in 1994.

Nutritional values per serving
(based on 8 servings):
calories: 178
fat: 7 g; 37% of calories
protein: 14 g; 31% of calories
carbohydrates: 14 g; 32% of calories

Spicy Black Bean Soup

Preparation time: 1½ hours

Although this recipe takes a little time to prepare, it's worth it. It is loaded with taste and is low in fat and very satisfying.

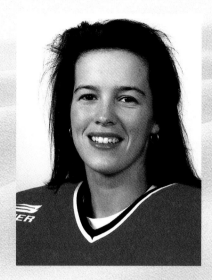

Cassie Campbell
W O M E N ' S
H O C K E Y

Cassie holds an honours degree in Sociology. She is currently a student in nutrition at the University of Guelph, where she was the Sportswoman of the Year in 1996. Originally from Richmond Hill, Ontario, the 25-year-old assistant captain has been a member of the national team since 1994. In her spare time, she enjoys soccer and basketball, and is a spokesperson for the HIP program, which is aimed at preventing young girls from smoking.

12 oz.	black beans, soaked	375 g
12 oz.	ham-hock bone	375 g
2 qts.	water or ham stock	2 L
2 oz.	sliced bacon	50 g
I	large onion	I
2	green peppers, chopped	2
2 cloves	garlic, chopped	2 cloves
I cup	orange juice	250 mL
2	bay leaves	2
I	chili pepper, whole	I
I tsp.	basil	5 mL
I tsp.	oregano	5 mL
I tsp.	salt	5 mL

Cook beans with ham bone for I hour or until beans are soft. Brown bacon in a frying pan. Add onion, green peppers and garlic, and sauté for a few minutes. Add to beans. Stir orange juice into frying pan, then pour into bean mixture. Add seasonings to beans, and simmer until vegetables are tender. Garnish with a dollop of sour cream or yogurt. Serves 12.

Nutritional values per serving
(based on 12 servings without garnish):
calories: 118
fat: 4 g; 31% of calories
protein: 8 g; 28% of calories
carbohydrates: 12 g; 40% of calories

Eddie's Chicken Feed

Preparation time: 20 minutes

I	chicken breast, skinned, boned and cut into bite-sized pieces	I
I tsp.	vegetable oil	5 mL
	romaine lettuce, torn into bite-sized pieces	
I0-I2	seedless grapes	I0-I2
I	carrot, chopped	I
I	apple, chopped	I
I Tbsp.	low-fat salad dressing	I5 mL
	herbed croutons	

Brown chicken in oil in frying pan. In a large bowl, combine chicken with lettuce, grapes and carrots. Chop and add the apple last so that it won't go brown. Top with low-fat salad dressing of your choice (poppy seed is good), and finish it off with herbed croutons. Serves I.

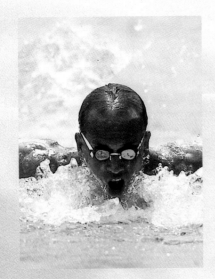

Eddie Parenti
S W I M M I N G

Eddie has been on the Canadian national swimming team for eight years. He participated in the 1992 and 1996 Olympics, and in the latter, he achieved his best times of 2:00.16 minutes in the 200-metre butterfly and :53.04 in the 100-metre butterfly. He has competed in the Commonwealth Games, the world swimming championships and seven Pan-Pacific Games as well as swimming for Stanford University between 1991 and 1995. Eddie was an All-American in 1991, 1992 and 1993 for the Stanford swimming team. He is now training with the Pacific Dolphins and working in Vancouver.

Nutritional values per serving
(based on 1 serving):
calories: 414
fat: 10 g; 21% of calories
protein: 33 g; 32% of calories
carbohydrates: 49 g; 47% of calories

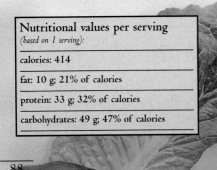

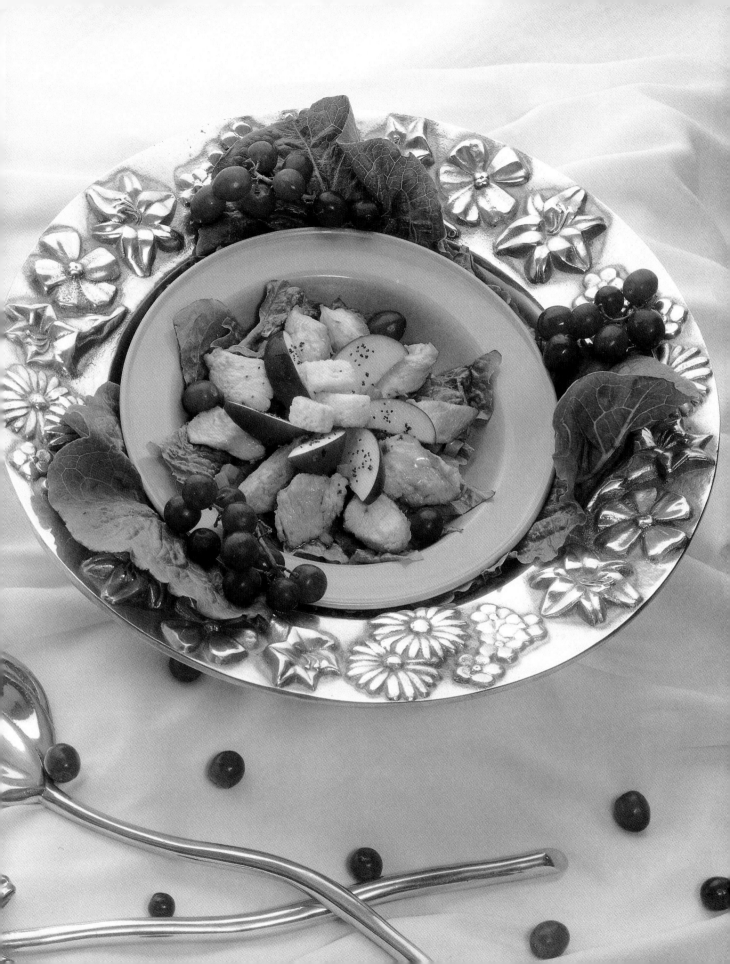

Feta Delight Salad

Preparation time: 15 minutes

This is Kelly's favourite recipe because it is quick to make, keeps well in the refrigerator and is easy to carry in a container for post-workout snacks. Best of all, it contains her favourite food: feta cheese. She usually eats this as a quick post-workout boost and as a healthy snack during the day when she is pressed for time. Other herbs and vegetables can be substituted for those listed.

2 cups	rotini or farfalle pasta	500 mL
10-12	fresh mushrooms, chopped	10-12
I each	green and red peppers, chopped	I each
4-5	Roma tomatoes, chopped	4-5
I Tbsp.	olive oil	15 mL
I Tbsp.	balsamic vinegar	15 mL
	salt and pepper	
	thyme	
	oregano	
	fresh parsley, chopped	
2 Tbsp.	feta cheese	25 mL

Cook pasta, and cool, then mix with vegetables. For dressing, combine oil, vinegar and seasonings to taste, pour over salad, mix well, and crumble feta cheese on top. Serves 4.

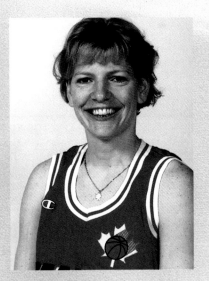

Kelly Boucher
BASKETBALL

Kelly joined the national team in 1988. She retired temporarily in 1991 but was lured back in 1993. She represented Canada at the 1989 and 1993 COPABA world qualification tournaments and was also a member of the Canadian team at the 1994 Goodwill Games in Russia and the 1994 world championships in Australia. The 1995 national women's team won the gold medal at the COPABA Olympic qualification tournament in Hamilton, Ontario. She averaged 28.6 points and 11 rebounds last season in Switzerland and is currently playing professional basketball in Germany.

Nutritional values per serving
(based on 4 servings):
calories: 281
fat: 6 g; 18% of calories
protein: 9 g; 13% of calories
carbohydrates: 49 g; 69% of calories

Kelly's Performance Eating Tip:

When pan-frying chicken, use lemon juice in a nonstick pan instead of oil. Substitute plain yogurt for mayonnaise and sour cream.

Apple-Avocado Salad

Preparation time: 15 minutes

2	avocados, sliced	2
2	apples, with skin, chopped	2
1 tsp.	Dijon mustard	5 mL
2 Tbsp.	lemon juice	25 mL
¼ cup	olive oil	125 mL
¼ cup	fresh parsley, chopped	125 mL
	salt and pepper	
¼ cup	toasted slivered almonds	125 mL

Place avocados and apples in a bowl. Combine mustard, lemon juice, oil, parsley and salt and pepper to taste. Mix well, and pour over fruit. Add almonds, and toss. Serves 4.

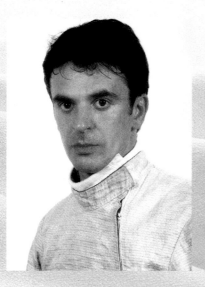

Jean-Paul Banos
FENCING

In the 1996 Olympics, Jean-Paul was the longest-standing team member, with 18 years to his credit. He holds more titles than any other Canadian fencer (24 senior, junior and team). Besides being very active in international sports himself, he is also technical and administrative director of the Fédération d'escrime du Québec and competition organizer and coach at the Brébeuf Club. In 1991, he was captain of the sabre team that made 6th at the world championships, the best ever Canadian showing, which assured qualification for the Barcelona Olympics.

Nutritional values per serving
(based on 4 servings):
calories: 426
fat: 34 g; 72% of calories
protein: 4 g; 4% of calories
carbohydrates: 26 g; 24% of calories

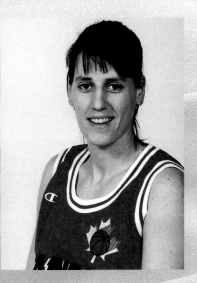

Shawna Molcak
B A S K E T B A L L

Shawna, who was born and raised in Cardston, Alberta, and attended the University of Lethbridge, has been active in many sports, both recreationally and at a competitive level. Basketball is her favourite, but she also enjoys golf and softball. The 1996 Olympics were her first. Shawna is currently playing professional basketball in Greece.

Caesar Salad

Preparation time: 20 minutes

This is Shawna's favourite peak-performance recipe because it tastes very good, is a bit spicy and provides an extra boost. Any time of day is good for this salad. Leftover dressing can be stored in the refrigerator for later use. It becomes spicier after it sits for a day or so.

I tsp.	pepper	5 mL
I tsp.	seasoned salt	5 mL
I tsp.	Tabasco sauce	5 mL
I tsp.	Worcestershire sauce	5 mL
I clove	garlic, crushed	I clove
I Tbsp.	fresh lemon juice	15 mL
2 Tbsp.	red wine vinegar	25 mL
6 Tbsp.	vegetable oil	75 mL
I	egg yolk	I
	romaine lettuce, torn into bite-sized pieces	
	croutons	
	Parmesan cheese	

Combine pepper and seasoned salt. Add Tabasco sauce and Worcestershire sauce, and mix well. Add garlic, lemon juice, vinegar, oil and egg yolk. Stir together until well blended. Pour dressing over lettuce, and add croutons and Parmesan cheese. Serves 4.

Nutritional values per serving
(based on 4 servings):
calories: 287
fat: 25 g; 80% of calories
protein: 4 g; 7% of calories
carbohydrates: 9 g; 13% of calories

Lean-and-Mean Caesar Salad

Preparation time: 15 minutes

Because Caesar salad can be heavy in fat and calories, Carrie created this lighter version. She normally eats it post-event or after a long day at the gym. She sometimes adds chicken to the salad. For a tangier flavour, balsamic vinegar can be substituted for cider vinegar.

I head	romaine lettuce, torn into bite-sized pieces	I head
	garlic- or Caesar-flavoured croutons	
I cup	low-fat yogurt	250 mL
¼ cup	extra-virgin olive oil	125 mL
¼ cup	cider vinegar	125 mL
2 cloves	garlic, crushed	2 cloves
	freshly ground black pepper	
	oregano	
	basil	
	cumin	
	dry mustard	
	dill	
	marjoram	
	seasoned salt	
	Worcestershire sauce	
	freshly grated Parmesan cheese	

Combine lettuce and croutons in a bowl. Place all remaining ingredients (seasonings to taste) except Parmesan cheese in a jar, and shake vigorously (use your throwing arm, and pretend you're throwing fastballs!). Pour dressing over top (you may not need the whole jar), and toss well. Sprinkle cheese on top, and toss again. Carrie likes to put a little more freshly ground pepper on top. Serves 4.

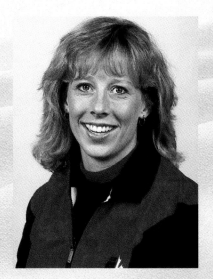

Carrie Flemmer
S O F T B A L L

Carrie, who is 29, was born in Stettler, Alberta, and raised in North Delta, British Columbia. She played for 17 years with the North Delta Minors, six years with the White Rock Renegades (the 1992 and 1993 national champions) and six years with the Canadian national team. She is the starting catcher for the Canadian women's national team, which placed 5th at the 1996 Olympic Games, won a silver medal at the national championships in Saskatoon and a gold medal at the Canada Cup in Surrey, British Columbia.

Nutritional values per serving
(based on 4 servings):
calories: 246
fat: 18 g; 67% of calories
protein: 7 g; 11% of calories
carbohydrates: 14 g; 22% of calories

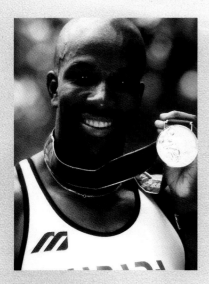

Donovan Bailey
R U N N I N G

Fans and critics alike have called Donovan "the world's fastest man". Since taking up racing in 1994, he has set new world records in both the 100 meter, and 50 meter indoor, as well as a Canadian record in the 4x100 relay. Born in Manchester, Jamaica, he now resides in Austin, Texas where he is a member of the South Regional Phoenix Track Club.

Tangy Salad Dressing

Preparation time: 10 minutes

Served over a salad, this dressing is a great part of a light peak-performance lunch.

2 tsp.	cornstarch	10 mL
1 tsp.	hot mustard	5 mL
1 tsp.	paprika	5 mL
¼ tsp.	ground white peppercorns	1 mL
¼ tsp.	granulated garlic	1 mL
½ cup	cold water	125 mL
¼ cup	red wine	50 mL
3 Tbsp.	sugar	40 mL
2 Tbsp.	olive oil	25 mL
¼ tsp.	salt	1 mL

Simmer all ingredients in a saucepan for 1 minute. Taste, and add more sugar if too tart or red wine if too sweet. Cool for at least 10 minutes before serving, preferably in the refrigerator. Makes 1 cup.

Nutritional values per serving
(based on 6 servings):

calories: 79

fat: 5 g; 52% of calories

protein: 0 g; 1% of calories

carbohydrates: 8 g; 39% of calories

Sesame Noodles

Preparation time: 25 minutes

This dish is a great-tasting source of carbohydrates and energy, good during training season or for a pre-race meal. Easy to make, it can be served hot or chilled as an accompaniment to spicy pork, beef or chicken. To serve the noodles chilled, place them in a bowl, cool to room temperature, cover, and refrigerate for an hour.

1 lb.	noodles	500 g
3 Tbsp.	sesame seeds	40 mL
5	green onions, green parts only, chopped	5
1 Tbsp.	peanut oil	15 mL
2 Tbsp.	Chinese sesame oil	25 mL
1 Tbsp.	Chinese 5-spice powder	15 mL
	salt and pepper	
	roasted peanuts (optional)	

In a large pot of water, boil noodles for 6-8 minutes or until tender. Drain, rinse under cool water, and drain again. In a small skillet over medium heat, toast the sesame seeds, stirring continuously, until they are fragrant and golden; set aside. Place green onions in a saucepan set over boiling water. Cook over medium-high heat for 4 minutes, then remove the pan from the heat. Place peanut oil and 1 Tbsp. sesame oil in a wok, and heat over high heat until the oils are very hot. Add green onions, and stir-fry for 1 minute. Add 5-spice powder and noodles, and stir-fry until heated through. Add the remaining sesame oil and the sesame seeds. Season to taste with salt and pepper. Place noodles in a serving dish, and garnish with roasted peanuts if desired. Serves 5.

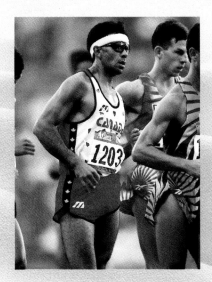

Arturo Huerta
R A C E W A L K I N G

Arturo began athletics because he wanted something that would give him a sense of direction while having fun and meeting good people at the same time. He chose racewalking because it is very hard to master technically, needing both endurance and good coordination. His goal is to make the medal podium in the world championships, the World Cup races or the Olympic Games. In 1996, he won the Canadian nationals and represented Canada in Atlanta. Also in 1996, he achieved a personal best (1:22:51) in the 20-km race at Washington, D.C.

Nutritional values per serving
(based on 5 servings; without peanuts):
calories: 458
fat: 15 g; 30% of calories
protein: 14 g; 13% of calories
carbohydrates: 66 g; 59% of calories

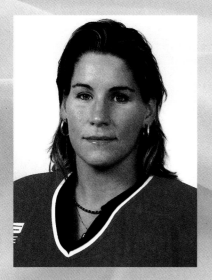

Lori Dupuis
WOMEN'S HOCKEY

Although Lori has only been a member of the national team since 1995, she has distinguished herself as a valuable player in that time. She has competed twice in the Pacific Rim Chamionships (winning gold both times), twice in the Three Nations Cup (one gold and one silver) and won a gold at the Worlds in 1997. Lori studies French and geography at the University of Toronto and enjoys a variety of sports, travelling and reading.

Saffron Rice

Preparation time: 30 minutes

This one is one of Lori's favourite meals. It is low in fat, easy to prepare and tastes wonferful.

2 tsp.	vegetable oil	10 mL
6	whole cloves	6
¼ tsp.	ground cinnamon	1 mL
1 tsp.	salt	5 mL
¼ tsp.	saffron	1 mL
1½ cups	long-grain rice	375 mL
2¼ cups	chicken stock	550 mL
2 tsp.	18% table cream	10 mL

Heat oil in saucepan, add seasonings, and sauté for 30 seconds. Add rice, and sauté for 1 minute or until rice is coated with oil. Add stock, and bring to a simmer, cover, and cook for 15-20 minutes. Stir in cream. Let rest for 5 minutes, then fluff rice just before serving. Garnish with sliced apples or pears. Serves 6.

Nutritional values per serving
(based on 6 servings):
calories: 203
fat: 3 g; 13% of calories
protein: 4 g; 8% of calories
carbohydrates: 40 g; 79% of calories

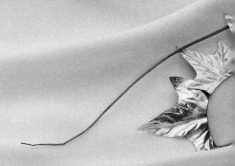

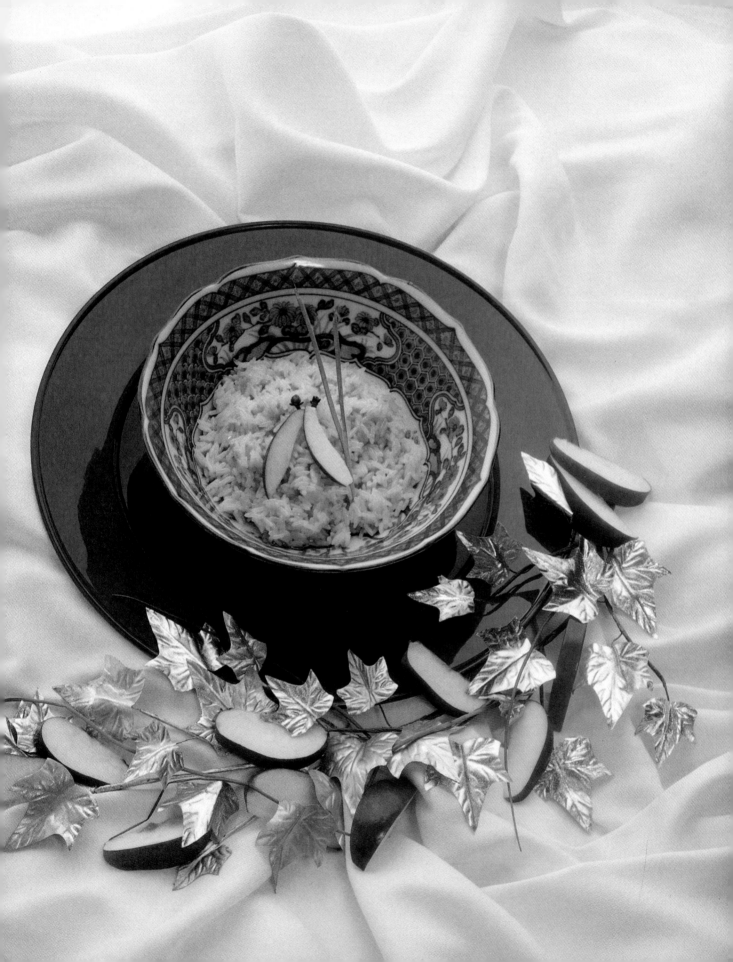

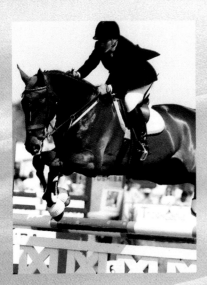

Linda Southern Heathcott
EQUESTRIAN

Linda, who began her riding career at age eight, is well known on the Canadian show-jumping circuit. In 1981, she was Canadian Junior Jumper Champion and represented Alberta on the Continental Young Riders Team, which won the team silver medal in both 1982 and 1983. In 1991, she was 2nd in the Canadian championships and, in 1993, won the overall Canadian team trials. In 1996, she competed in her first Olympics.

Linda's Rice Dish

Preparation time: 2½ hours

A real energy food without being heavy, this is Linda's favourite peak-performance dish. She normally eats it the evening before an event. It is good served with fish. The casserole can be prepared the day before and baked just before serving.

6 oz.	wild rice	170 g
I cup	boiling water	250 mL
I cup	sliced mushrooms	250 mL
I Tbsp.	vegetable oil	15 mL
½ cup	butter or margarine	125 mL
I cup	grated cheddar cheese	250 mL
I tsp.	salt	5 mL
I cup	canned tomatoes	250 mL

Place wild rice in a double boiler, cover with boiling water, and cook for I hour or until tender. Meanwhile, sauté mushrooms in oil. Drain rice if necessary, and add mushrooms and the remaining ingredients. Place in a 2-qt. (2 L) buttered casserole, and bake for I hour at 350°F (180°C). Serves 6 as a side dish.

Nutritional values per serving
(based on 6 servings):
calories: 351
fat: 24 g; 62% of calories
protein: 10 g; 11% of calories
carbohydrates: 23 g; 27% of calories

Hominy Grits With Cheddar Cheese

Preparation time: 30 minutes

This tasty dish is quick and easy to prepare. Try serving it with a salad for a complete meal.

2 cups	water	500 mL
I cup	ground hominy grits (quick cooking)	250 mL
½ cup	diced onions	125 mL
¼ tsp.	salt	1 mL
I tsp.	Tabasco sauce	5 mL
4 oz.	grated cheddar cheese	125 mL
2 oz.	butter	50 g
I	medium egg	I

Bring water to a boil, add grits and onions, and simmer for 5 minutes.

Add seasonings, cheese, butter and egg, and blend well. Pour into a lightly greased pan, and bake in a preheated 375°F (190°C) oven for 20 minutes. Serves 4.

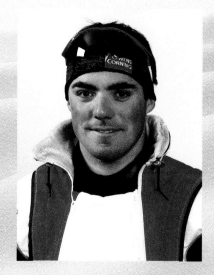

Nicolas Fontaine
FREESTYLE SKIING

This bilingual native of Magog, Quebec says of his successes, "I owe it all to hard work in the off-season, and experience." He has been a national team member since 1990, and is a three-time national aerials champion (1990, 1996, 1997). When he is not practising new jumps on the slopes, Nicolas enjoys tennis, mountain biking, golf, sailing, and water skiing.

Nutritional values per serving
(based on 4 servings):
calories: 391
fat: 23 g; 52% of calories
protein: 13 g; 13% of calories
carbohydrates: 34 g; 35% of calories

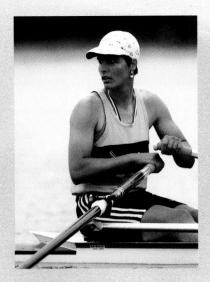

Diane O'Grady
R O W I N G

Diane, who is from North Bay, Ontario, began rowing competitively at the age of 21 when she was a student at Queen's University. Once she reached the elite level, she wondered how far she could go, a question that was answered when she made it to the 1996 Olympic Games. In 1995, Diane placed 1st in the 2x at the Pan American Games and 2nd in the 4x at the world championships, and in 1994, she placed first in 1x, 4x and 4- in the Canadian championships.

Mark's Famous Red Sauce

Preparation time: 20 minutes

This thick, flavourful sauce is good alone, with browned ground meat, on Chicken Parmesan, in lasagna or . . . well, lots of things! Diane usually has this dish for dinner during heavy training.

I	onion, chopped	I
I Tbsp.	olive oil	15 mL
28-oz. can	tomatoes, drained and chopped	796 mL
5½-oz. can	tomato paste	156 mL
I clove	garlic, minced	I clove
2 Tbsp.	basil	25 mL
I Tbsp.	oregano	15 mL
I tsp.	crushed rosemary	5 mL
2 Tbsp.	grated Parmesan cheese	25 mL

Sauté onion in oil over medium-high heat until translucent. Add tomatoes, and reduce heat to medium. Add tomato paste, garlic, basil, oregano and rosemary, and heat until mixture bubbles. Reduce heat to low, and stir in Parmesan cheese just before serving. Serve over pasta, with a little more Parmesan sprinkled on top. Serves 4.

Nutritional values per serving
(based on 4 servings; without pasta):

calories: 160

fat: 6 g; 31% of calories

protein: 5 g; 13% of calories

carbohydrates: 22 g; 56% of calories

Simple Barbecue Sauce

Preparation time: 10 minutes

This sauce is low in fat and so easy to prepare. Whether you are grilling beef, chicken, seafood or even vegetables, this is the perfect choice.

14-oz. can	plain tomato sauce	398 mL
1	medium onion, finely chopped	1
1 tsp.	Dijon mustard	5 mL
1 tsp.	Tabasco sauce	5 mL
½ cup	vinegar	125 mL
1 clove	garlic, crushed	1 clove
1 tsp.	paprika	5 mL
1 tsp.	Worcestershire sauce	5 mL
1 tsp.	sugar	5 mL
	salt and pepper	

Combine all ingredients in a saucepan, bring to a boil, and cook until preferred consistency is reached. Makes 2 cups.

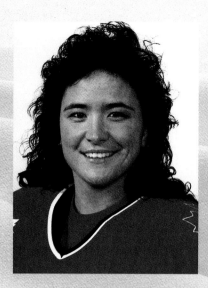

Vicky Sunohara
WOMEN'S HOCKEY

Vicky began her hockey career with Scarborough Girls and Boys Hockey in 1975, at the age of five. By the age of 13, she was the NCAA Championship Rookie of the Year. Since then, she has attained many awards, including a gold at the 1997 World Championships, scoring four goals and one assist in five games, and a gold at the 1996 Three-Nation's Cup. Vicky also distinguished herself at the World Championships in 1990, scoring six goals and three assists in five games.

Nutritional values per serving
(based on 8 servings):
calories: 35
fat: 0 g; 5% of calories
protein: 1 g; 12% of calories
carbohydrates: 7 g; 83% of calories

Avocado Salsa

Preparation time: 10 minutes

This is a great way to handle those "munchie attacks" that plague even athletes. Quick and easy to prepare, this dish is a perfect snack anytime.

1	medium onion, chopped	1
1 tsp.	vegetable oil	5 mL
3-4	tomatillos, roasted and peeled	3-4
2 cloves	garlic, crushed	2 cloves
2 tsp.	lemon juice	10 mL
1 tsp.	salt	5 mL
1 tsp.	pepper	5 mL
2	avocados, peeled and diced	2

Sauté onion in oil. Cut tomatillos in half, and add to onions. Add garlic, lemon juice, salt and pepper, and cook for 2 minutes. Cool, purée in food processor or blender, and mix with avocados. Makes 3 cups.

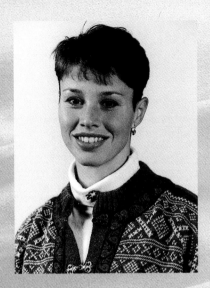

Catriona Le May Doan
SPEED SKATING

Catriona is not only an impressive skater, she is an award-winning all-around athlete. In 1993, she competed in the Canada Summer Games, and won two bronze medals and a silver in track and field. She has set world records in the 500 metre and 1500 metre, and a Canadian record in the 1000 metre. Born in 1970 in Saskatoon, Saskatchewan, Catriona is currently a student at the University of Calgary.

Nutritional values per serving
(based on 9 servings):

calories: 98

fat: 7 g; 68% of calories

protein: 1 g; 6% of calories

carbohydrates: 6 g; 26% of calories

Salmon and Almond Cheese Spread

Preparation time: 1¼ hours

Isabelle is a fan of restaurants, and knows how important presentation is. Placed on a fancy plate and surrounded by elegant crackers, this dish is an attractive addition to any buffet.

14-oz. can	salmon, drained and bones removed	398 mL
1 tsp.	chopped green onion	5 mL
¼ tsp.	salt	1 mL
1 tsp.	lemon juice	5 mL
1 tsp.	chopped dill	5 mL
8 oz.	cream cheese, softened	250 g
3 oz.	plain yogurt	75 g
3 oz.	slivered almonds, toasted	75 g

Mix salmon, onions and seasonings together. Fold in cream cheese and yogurt until blended. Form into a ball, and roll in almonds. Refrigerate for 1 hour. If you are making this a day ahead, cover with plastic wrap. Serve with your favourite crackers.

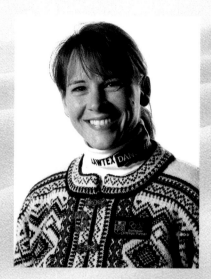

Isabelle Charest
S P E E D   S K A T I N G

Isabelle began her skating career as a figure skater, but eventually found speed skating more to her liking. Since joining the national team in 1988, she has competed in numerous World and World Team Championships. In 1996, she took the 500 World Crown, and entered the 1997-98 season as the world record holder in that event. Isabelle enjoys music and movies and credits teammate Natalie Lambert as her greatest encouragement and inspiration.

Nutritional values per serving
(based on 24 servings):
calories: 73
fat: 6 g; 73% of calories
protein: 4 g; 21% of calories
carbohydrates: 1 g; 6% of calories

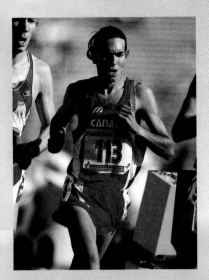

Peter Fonseca
R U N N I N G

When Peter crossed the finish line in 3rd place at the 1990 Los Angeles Marathon, everyone wondered who the kid was who finished 12 seconds behind the winner. In Atlanta, he was 21st in a field of 126. Born in Lisbon, Portugal, but raised in Toronto, Peter entered the world of competitive track and field at the relatively late age of 15, when he ran in a local road race. After training on the roads and trails of Toronto, he earned a scholarship to the University of Oregon, where he was named an All-American in 1990. His personal best is 2:11:34, and he has ranked 1st in Canada in four of the last six years.

Nutritional values per serving
(based on 4 servings):

calories: 651	
fat: 40 g; 55% of calories	
protein: 32 g; 20% of calories	
carbohydrates: 41 g; 25% of calories	

Deluxe Fajita Nachos

Preparation time: 30 minutes

Peter loves finger foods, and for him, nachos are the best kind, conjuring up memories of great times with fantastic friends. He usually has nachos after events or at parties. Sliced jalapeño peppers will spice up the dish; you can also use different meats.

2½ cups	cooked, shredded chicken	625 mL
1-oz. pkg.	fajita seasoning	30 g
⅓ cup	water	75 mL
8 oz.	tortilla chips	250 g
1 cup	grated Monterey jack cheese	250 mL
1¼ cups	grated cheddar cheese	375 mL
1	large tomato, chopped	1
¼ cup	sliced ripe olives	50 mL
¼ cup	sliced green onions	50 mL
	salsa	

In a skillet over medium heat, combine chicken, fajita seasoning and water. Bring to a boil, then reduce heat, and simmer for 3 minutes. Arrange tortilla chips on a large ovenproof platter, and top with chicken mixture and cheeses. Place under broiler to melt cheese. Top with tomato, olives, green onions and salsa to taste. Serves 4.

Peter's Performance Eating Tip:

Although I love nachos and could eat them almost every day, I am a great believer in moderation and variety.

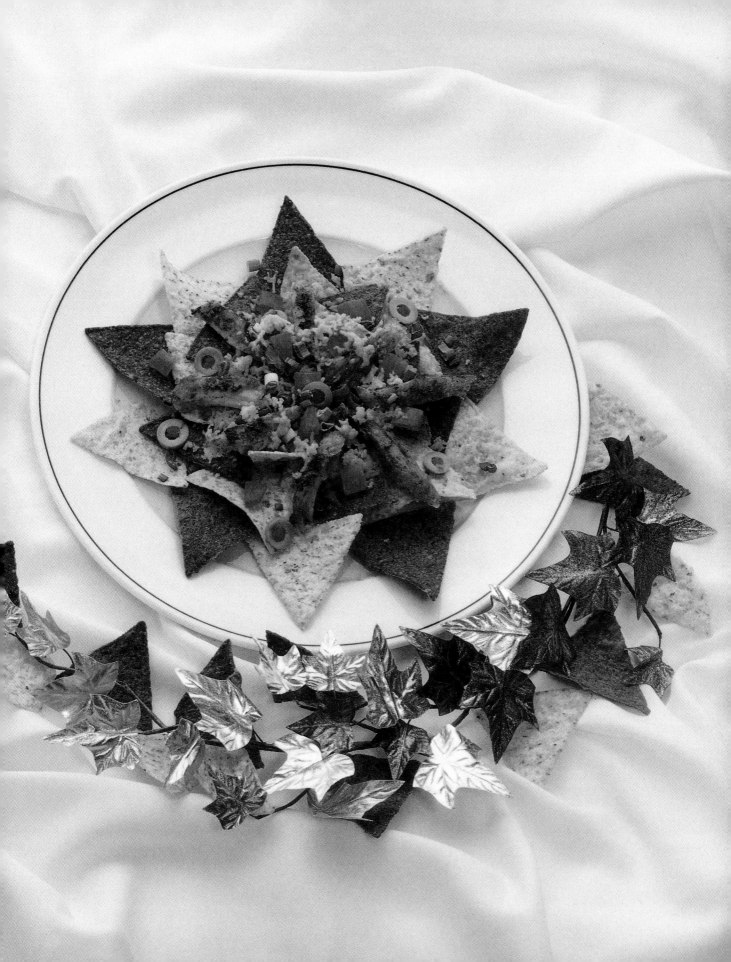

Sweet Success

Winner's Bars

Preparation time: 45 minutes

Martine finds that these bars give her all the energy she needs to win a race. She normally eats them between preliminaries and finals—exactly three hours before finals.

3 cups	oatmeal	750 mL
1 cup	sunflower seeds	250 mL
1 cup	raisins	250 mL
½ cup	melted butter	125 mL
1 cup	rice cereal	250 mL
1¼ cups	low-fat evaporated milk	300 mL
1 cup	chocolate chips	250 mL

Preheat oven to 325°F (160°C). Mix all ingredients together, and press into a 9-x-13-inch (3 L) baking tin, and bake for 20-25 minutes. Makes 36 bars.

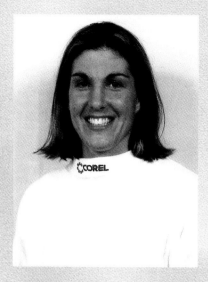

Martine Dessureault
S W I M M I N G

A full-time student of computing sciences at the Université du Québec à Montréal, Martine is a member of the Montréal-Nord swimming club. A member of the national team since 1995 and of the 1996 Olympic team, she placed 1st in the 50-metre at the Olympic trials and 26th in the Olympic Games. She has held number-one ranking in Quebec since 1994.

Nutritional values per bar
(based on 36 bars):
calories: 126
fat: 7 g; 51% of calories
protein: 3 g; 9% of calories
carbohydrates: 13 g; 40% of calories

Martine's Performance Eating Tip:

Eat plenty of pasta the week before a competition.

Energy Bars

Preparation time: 1¼ hours

Josée's favourite snack, these bars are an excellent source of energy and easy to carry.

¼ cup	margarine or butter	50 mL
⅓ cup	brown sugar	75 mL
½ cup	corn syrup	125 mL
½ tsp.	vanilla	2 mL
½ cup	dates	125 mL
½ cup	dried apricots	125 mL
½ cup	chopped almonds	125 mL
½ Tbsp.	grated orange peel	8 mL
6 cups	corn flakes	1.5 L

In a saucepan over low heat, melt margarine, then add sugar, corn syrup, vanilla, dates, apricots, almonds and orange peel. Gently mix in corn flakes. Press mixture into a 9-x-9-inch (2.5 L) casserole dish, and cool in refrigerator for 1 hour. Makes 24 bars.

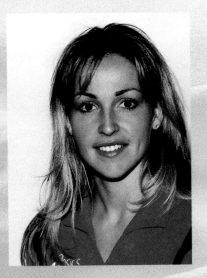

Josée Corbeil
V O L L E Y B A L L

Josée, who has been a member of the national team since 1993, lives in Winnipeg, Manitoba, where she is a physical education student. She enjoys aerobics, reading, beach volleyball and sewing. In 1995, she was the bronze medallist at the Pan American Games and now has her sights set on the 2000 Olympics in Sydney.

Nutritional values per bar
(based on 24 bars):
calories: 118
fat: 4 g; 27% of calories
protein: 1 g; 5% of calories
carbohydrates: 20 g; 68% of calories

Josée's Performance Eating Tip:

Eat several servings of fruits and vegetables every day.

Benoît's Bars

Preparation time: 40 minutes

While this is not Benoît's peak-performance food, the bars are a tasty, healthful snack that he usually eats before or after a workout.

3 cups	oatmeal	750 mL
1 cup	carob chips	250 mL
½ cup	dried fruit	125 mL
½ cup	chopped nuts	125 mL
½ cup	sunflower oil	125 mL
1½ cups	low-fat evaporated milk	375 mL

Preheat oven to 375°F (190°C). Combine dry ingredients in a bowl. In a separate bowl, mix oil and milk together, then add to dry ingredients. Pour into a 9-x-13-inch (3 L) pan, and bake for 25 minutes. Cool before cutting into bars. Makes 36 bars.

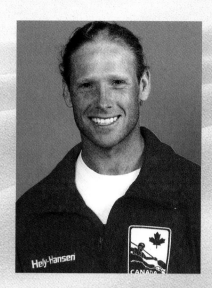

Benoît Gauthier
CANOEING

Benoît has competed in the Canadian nationals in slalom canoe since 1989. In 1993, he and François Letourneau began competing together and have won at the nationals for three years running. They came up with strong performances in 1996 at both the Olympics in Atlanta and the World Cup in Spain.

Nutritional values per bar
(based on 36 bars):
calories: 86
fat: 5 g; 50% of calories
protein: 2 g; 10% of calories
carbohydrates: 9 g; 40% of calories

Benoît's Performance Eating Tip:

The old adage "you are what you eat" is true. Allow only good food into your system, add exercise, and voilà, you have the recipe for life!

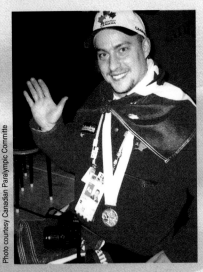

Daniel Labrie
SLEDGE HOCKEY

Daniel has been a competitor in sledge hockey since 1992, and has won numerous gold and silver medals at the national level. He joined Canada's National Sledge Hockey team in 1997 and has brought to the team a powerful blend of courage and determination. When not playing sledge hockey, Daniel spends his time pursuing a wide variety of interests: scuba diving, football, alpine skiing and cycling, to name a few.

Granola Bars

Preparation time: 45 minutes

This delicious snack is sure to raise your energy level. Take it along for that much needed boost, any time of the day.

3 cups	rolled oats	750 mL
1 cup	chopped nuts	250 mL
1 cup	dates, or chopped dried fruit	250 mL
1 cup	sunflower seeds	250 mL
1 cup	semi-sweet chocolate chips (optional)	250 mL
1 can	condensed milk	1 can
½ cup	butter, melted	125 mL

Preheat oven to 325°F (160°C). Line a jellyroll pan with foil and grease it. In a large mixing bowl, combine all ingredients, and mix well. Press evenly into prepared pan. Bake for 25-30 minutes, or until golden brown. Cool slightly, remove from pan, and peel off foil. Cut into bars. Store at room temperature, loosely covered. Makes 36 bars.

Nutritional values per serving
(based on 12 servings):
calories: 504
fat: 29 g; 51% of calories
protein: 11 g; 8% of calories
carbohydrates: 51 g; 40% of calories

Bran and Oatmeal Squares

Preparation time: 30 minutes

"A good high-fibre post-event snack," says Alan.

1¾ cups	all-bran cereal	400 mL
1¾ cups	quick-cooking rolled oats	400 mL
¾ cup	all-purpose flour	150 mL
1 cup	coconut	250 mL
¾ cup	brown sugar	150 mL
¾ cup	butter	150 mL
2 Tbsp.	corn syrup	25 mL
1 tsp.	baking soda	5 mL

Preheat oven to 350°F (180°C). Combine bran, oats, flour and coconut in a bowl. Heat sugar, butter and corn syrup over medium heat until the mixture boils, stirring constantly. Remove from heat, and stir in baking soda. Stir into cereal mixture, and mix well. Press into shallow, greased 9-x-13-inch (3 L) baking pan, and bake for 12-15 minutes. Makes 40 squares.

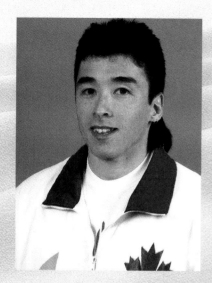

Alan Nolet
G Y M N A S T I C S

Alan has been a member of the Canadian national team since 1986. In the 1990 Commonwealth Games, he placed 1st in horizontal bars and 2nd in both floor and all around, and in 1994, he made a 1st in horizontal bars and a 3rd in floor. In the Pan American Games in 1995, he placed 4th in both rings and parallel bars, and his team placed 3rd. Alan, who lives in Hamilton, Ontario, enjoys fishing, golf, hockey and horseback riding.

Nutritional values per square
(based on 40 squares):
calories: 83
fat: 5 g; 49% of calories
protein: 1 g; 5% of calories
carbohydrates: 9 g; 46% of calories

Alan's Performance Eating Tip:

For a healthy diet, eat everything in moderation.

Carbo Cakes

Preparation time: 1 hour

Almost a complete meal, carbo cakes are an excellent source of carbohydrates. Jacques finds them especially good during and immediately after an event to replenish glycogen stores.

1 cup	rice or semolina	250 mL
4 cups	2% milk	1 L
¼ cup	raisins	50 mL
¾ cup	sugar	150 mL
4	eggs	4
¼ cup	butter	50 mL
2 tsp.	vanilla	10 mL

Preheat oven to 350°F (180°C). Boil rice in water for 3 minutes, drain, then add milk and raisins. Cook over medium heat, stirring occasionally, for 5 minutes. Mix in sugar, eggs, butter and vanilla, and cook, stirring, for another 5 minutes. Pour into a lightly greased loaf pan, and bake in oven for 30 minutes, or until a knife inserted in the centre comes out clean. Makes 8 cakes.

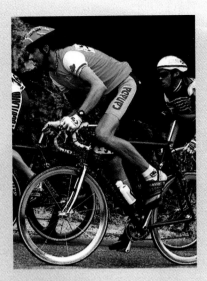

Jacques Landry
C Y C L I N G

Jacques was born in Saskatchewan and currently resides in Quebec. He excels in road racing, one of the most demanding cardiovascular sports. He has been a member of the Canadian national team since 1992, and his record to date includes 3rd place in Paris, a stage win in the Tour du Nord Izère (4th overall) and 6th at the Tour du Granitier Breton time trial (12th overall). In the 1995 Canadian championships, he placed 2nd in the individual time trials, and at the Olympic trials in 1996, he earned 3rd place.

Nutritional values per serving
(based on 8 cakes):
calories: 318
fat: 11 g; 31% of calories
protein: 9 g; 11% of calories
carbohydrates: 46 g; 58% of calories

Orange Sugar Cookies

Preparation time: 30 minutes

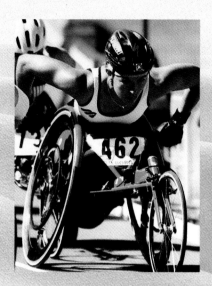

I cup	chilled butter, cut into I-inch (2.5 cm) cubes	250 mL
½ cup	sugar	125 mL
I Tbsp.	orange juice concentrate or orange liqueur	15 mL
I½ tsp.	orange zest	7 mL
I½ tsp.	lemon zest	7 mL
I tsp.	vanilla	5 mL
I½ cups	presifted self-rising flour	375 mL
4	medium seedless oranges, sectioned and patted dry	4

Chantal Petitclerc
W H E E L C H A I R A T H L E T I C S

Originally from Ste.-Foy, Quebec, Chantal has set new Canadian records in the 100, 200, 400, 800 and 1500 metre events. Widely recognized for her regular television appearances with Lotto Québec, Chantal also finds the time in her rigorous training schedule to be a role model. She is the honorary chair of the "Women's March Against Poverty", and is one of only four athletes with a disability chosen to receive a MetLife bursary.

Preheat oven to 350°F (180°C). Place butter and sugar in a food processor, and mix until smooth. Add orange juice concentrate, zests and vanilla, and mix. Add flour, and mix until dough is lightly blended. Do not overmix. Place in a piping bag with a plain tip, and pipe onto a lightly floured surface. Cut into I-inch (2.5 cm) pieces, roll into balls, and place on greased cookie sheet. Lightly press an orange section onto the top of each one. Bake for about 10 minutes or until lightly browned. Remove from oven, and let stand for 10 minutes. Makes 2 dozen cookies.

Nutritional values per serving
(based on 24 servings):
calories: 127
fat: 8 g; 55% of calories
protein: 1 g; 4% of calories
carbohydrates: 13 g; 41 % of calories

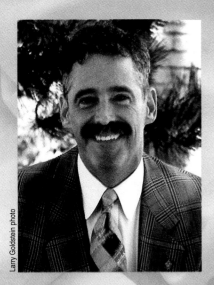

Larry Goldstein photo

Martin Glynn
BOBSLEIGH

Besides representing Canada as the pilot in the four-man bobsleigh event in 1980, Martin distinguished himself in many other areas. He spent six years in law enforcement, first with the Montreal Police Department, then with the RCMP. Since 1991, he has launched fund raising and awareness building initiatives benefiting the COA, education programs, Canadian unity, and UNICEF.

Martin continues to pursue athletic excellence, and has participated in 12 marathons, including the 100th running of the Boston Marathon. He is a sought after public speaker, and marketing professional.

Nutritional values per serving *(based on 48 servings):*		
calories: 40		
fat: 2g; 45% of calories		
protein: 0g; 4% of calories		
carbohydrates: 5g; 51% of calories		

Cinnamon Ginger Snaps
Preparation time: 45 minutes

Low in fat, yet brimming with flavour, these cookies are an excellent treat for any time of the day.

¼ cup	butter	50 mL
½ cup	molasses	125 mL
½ tsp.	baking soda	2 mL
1½ tsp.	warm water	7 mL
1¼ cups	all-purpose flour	300 mL
¼ tsp.	ground cloves	1 mL
½ tsp.	ground ginger	2 mL
2 tsp.	cinnamon	10 mL
1 tsp.	brown sugar	5 mL

Preheat oven to 350°F (180°C). In a heavy saucepan, gently melt butter, then add molasses, and simmer for a few minutes, stirring with a wooden spoon. Remove from heat, and let cool. In a stainless-steel bowl, whisk baking soda and warm water together, then add to butter mixture. In another bowl, mix flour, seasonings and brown sugar, then slowly stir in molasses mixture. Mix until well-blended, but do not overmix. Roll into cylinder, wrap in plastic wrap, and chill for 30 minutes. Cut into ⅛ inch (3 mm) slices, and bake for 6-7 minutes. Makes 3-4 dozen cookies.

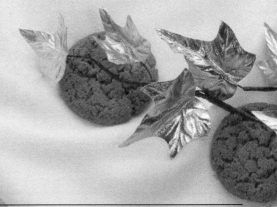

Martin's Performance Tip
Olympians are ordinary people who do extraordinary things, on a continual basis.

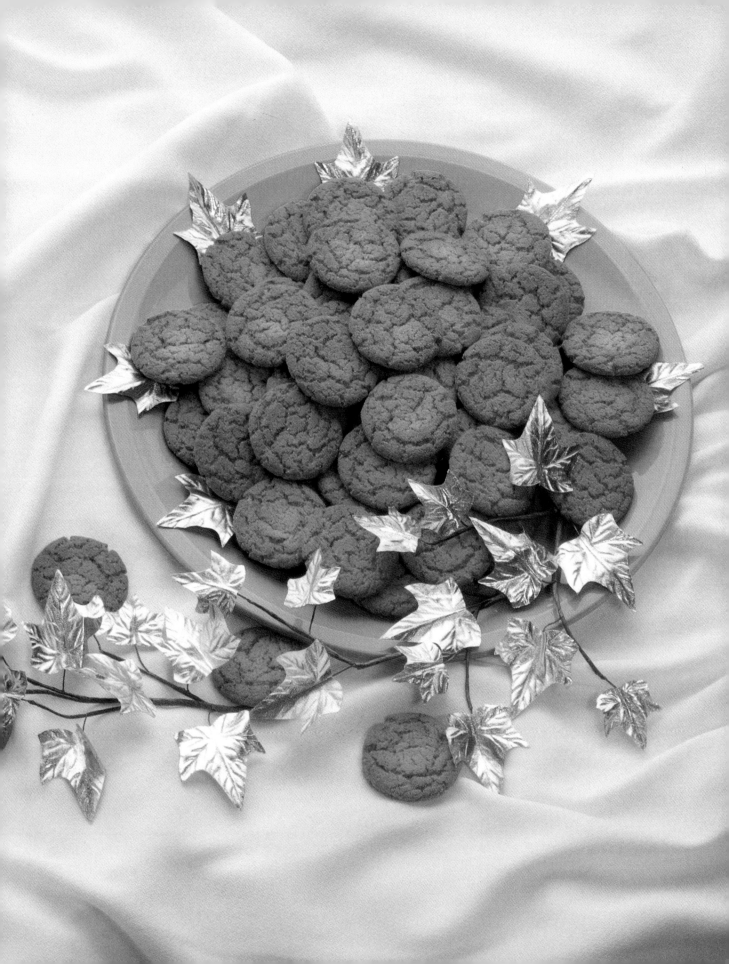

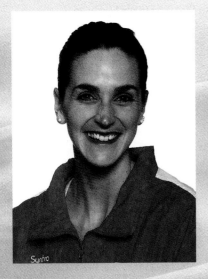

Sylvie Fréchette
SYNCHRONIZED SWIMMING

Sylvie took her first swimming lesson at the age of seven. In 1986 and 1990, she won gold at the Commonwealth Games. In 1991 she set a new world mark by scoring seven perfect 10s.

A judging error at the Barcelona Olympics cost her a gold medal. But after a lengthy review process, the IOC presented Sylvie with her gold medal in December 1993, in an official ceremony organized in her honour at the Montreal Forum and telecast live across Canada.

After almost two years of retirement from sports, Sylvie returned to training and won a silver medal in 1996.

Nutritional values per cookie (based on 60 cookies):
calories: 60
fat: 3 g; 45% of calories
protein: 1 g; 5% of calories
carbohydrates: 7 g; 50% of calories

Chocolate Chip Cookies

Preparation time: 30 minutes

These cookies are Sylvie's reward after a good performance.

½ cup	softened butter	125 mL
½ cup	white sugar	125 mL
½ cup	brown sugar	125 mL
2	large eggs	2
1 tsp.	vanilla	5 mL
2 cups	all-purpose flour	500 mL
1 tsp.	baking soda	5 mL
½ tsp.	salt	2 mL
½ cup	chocolate chips	125 mL

Preheat oven to 375°F (190°C). Cream together butter and sugars. Mix in eggs one at a time, then add vanilla. Sift together flour, baking soda and salt. Gradually add to creamed mixture, then fold in chocolate chips. Drop from a teaspoon onto a lightly greased cookie sheet, and bake for 10-12 minutes. Makes about 5 dozen cookies.

Sylvie's Performance Eating Tip:

Pasta is a must for an athlete, especially before an event.

The Officially Approved "Glycogen Window" Chocolate Chip Cookie

Preparation time: 30 minutes

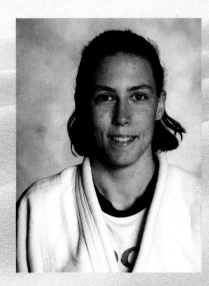

Carolyne Lepage
JUDO

Carolyne is from Montreal, where she lives and trains at the Club de Judo Varennes. In 1994 and 1995, she was Canadian senior champion in the 48-kg division, and in 1994, she placed 3rd at the Pan American championships and 2nd in the Pan American Games.

Judo is a weight-category sport, so Carolyne has to keep to a strict diet — a challenge because of her sweet tooth. But she finds that timing her cookie consumption according to the glycogen-window formula allows her to keep her weight in check, improve muscle rest and recovery rates and satisfy her sweet tooth. Isn't science wonderful?

½ cup	butter	125 mL
¾ cup	brown sugar	150 mL
¼ cup	egg substitute	50 mL
I tsp.	vanilla	5 mL
1¼ cups	all-purpose flour	300 mL
I tsp.	baking soda	5 mL
I cup	semisweet chocolate chips	250 mL

Preheat oven to 375°F (190°C). In a food processor, mix butter, sugar, egg substitute and vanilla. Add flour and baking soda, and mix again. Place the mixture in a large bowl, and fold in chocolate chips. With a teaspoon, drop looney-sized dollops of cookie dough I inch apart on a nonstick cookie sheet. For chewy cookies, bake for 7 minutes, and immediately move them from the cookie sheet to a cooling rack to prevent further cooking; for crunchier cookies, bake for 10 minutes. Makes about 4 dozen cookies.

Nutritional values per cookie
(based on 48 cookies):

calories: 57	
fat: 3 g; 51% of calories	
protein: 1 g; 4% of calories	
carbohydrates: 6 g; 45% of calories	

The Glycogen Window

Using the glycogen window, athletes can avoid the normal effects of eating sugars and fats (insulin surges, stimulation of fat-storage mechanisms and decreased mental alertness) by converting them directly into the energy needed after training. Here's how it works:
After a training session, the muscles have exhausted their store of glycogen—which is their energy source—and are hungry for glucose (the glycogen building block). At this stage, which is called the glycogen window, the body will greedily consume glucose and convert it directly into productive glycogen, speeding muscle recovery and bypassing the usual effects of high sugar intake.

Spinnaker Sweet Buns

Preparation time: 1½ hours

Tine likes these buns because they taste so good. "Try them with cheese, jam or berries," she says. She normally eats them between races because they're light and easy to carry.

10 Tbsp.	margarine	150 mL
2¾ cups	skim milk	650 mL
¾ cup	sugar	150 mL
1½ oz.	active dry yeast	50 g
6 cups	all-purpose flour	1.5 L
1 tsp.	ground cardamom	5 mL
½ cup	raisins	125 mL

Melt margarine, add milk, and warm the mixture until lukewarm. Combine all dry ingredients in a separate bowl. Add the wet ingredients to the dry. Let stand in warm area without air circulation for 1 hour. Preheat oven to 350°F (180°C). Knead the dough well, adding raisins (more if desired) while kneading. Form dough into 30 slightly flattened balls, place on greased cookie sheet, and bake for 10-12 minutes. Makes 30 buns.

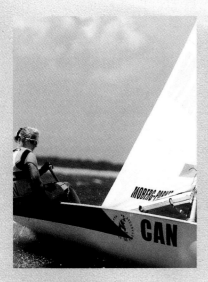

Tine Moberg-Parker
Y A C H T I N G

Tine started sailing at age six and went to her first world Optimist championship when she was 12. She was a member of Norway's national sailing team from 1989 to 1993. During that time, she came to Canada to learn English and later to attend Simon Fraser University. In her five years with the Norwegian team, Tine chalked up five top-10 finishes (Europe class) at the world championships. In 1991, she won the world title in Los Angeles. After getting her release from the Norwegian Sailing Federation, she joined the Canadian national team in 1994.

Nutritional values per bun
(based on 30 buns):
calories: 170
fat: 5 g; 26% of calories
protein: 4 g; 10% of calories
carbohydrates: 27 g; 64% of calories

Tine's Performance Eating Tip:

Use applesauce as a partial substitute for butter and sugar.

Raisin Loaf

Preparation time: 1 hour

This is a terrific high-protein snack for any time of the day.

2 cups	flour	500 mL
½ tsp.	salt	2 mL
3 tsp.	baking powder	15 mL
¾ cup	sugar	150 mL
1 cup	raisins	250 mL
1 cup	milk	250 mL
2 Tbsp.	corn syrup	25 mL

Preheat oven to 350°F (180°C). Sift flour, salt, and baking powder into a bowl, then mix in sugar and raisins. Heat milk and syrup together until blended but not hot. Make a well in the centre of the dry ingredients, and pour in the liquid. Stir quickly until all the mixture is dampened. Turn into a greased 8-inch loaf tin and bake for 40-45 minutes.

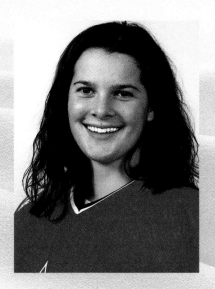

Jennifer Botterill
WOMEN'S HOCKEY

A student at the University of Calgary, Jennifer studies kinesiology, both academically and practically. She was proclaimed Athlete of the Year in high school and has competed in soccer and track and field. Jennifer also played in the Junior National Baseball Championships, and is a provincial badminton champion (Manitoba). At 18, she is the youngest member of Team Canada.

Nutritional values per serving
(based on 12 servings):

calories: 191

fat: 1 g; 4% of calories

protein: 3 g; 7% of calories

carbohydrates: 42 g; 89% of calories

François's Rice Pudding

Preparation time: 15 minutes

François finds rice pudding nutritious, simple to make and easy to digest. Tasty hot or cold, it makes a good dessert — or even breakfast.

2	eggs	2
2 Tbsp.	cornstarch	25 mL
2 cups	2% milk	500 mL
½ cup	sugar	125 mL
I tsp.	vanilla	5 mL
I tsp.	butter	5 mL
2 cups	cooked rice	500 mL
¼ cup	raisins	50 mL
	nutmeg	

In a bowl, whisk together eggs, cornstarch and milk, mixing well to remove any lumps. Add sugar and vanilla, then cook over medium heat, stirring constantly, until mixture thickens. Remove from heat, and stir in butter and rice, then raisins and nutmeg to taste. Serves 4.

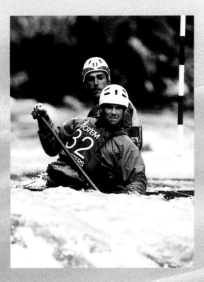

François Letourneau
CANOEING

François has competed in slalom canoe in the Canadian nationals since 1989. In 1993, he and Benoît Gauthier began competing together and have won at the nationals for three years running. They came up with strong performances in 1996 at both the Olympics in Atlanta and the World Cup in Spain.

Nutritional values per serving
(based on 4 servings):
calories: 384
fat: 6 g; 14% of calories
protein: 10 g; 11% of calories
carbohydrates: 72 g; 75% of calories

Hanger's Bread Pudding

Preparation time: 2½ hours

Clara likes this pudding because it is low-fat, high-carbohydrate, great-tasting, simple and inexpensive. She normally has it for breakfast or a snack wrapped up to eat during a long training ride. (Michael Barry's recipe)

I loaf	stale French bread	I loaf
I cup	raisins	250 mL
4 cups	2% milk	I L
3	eggs	3
I cup	sugar	250 mL
2 Tbsp.	vanilla	25 mL

Cut bread into small pieces, and place in a large bowl with raisins. Pour milk over them, and let stand for I hour. Preheat oven to 325°F (160°C). In a separate bowl, beat eggs, then mix in sugar and vanilla. Combine gently with bread mixture, then pour into a nonstick or greased 9-x-13-inch (3 L) baking pan. Bake for 1½ hours or until brown. Serve hot or cold, plain or with custard or ice cream. Serves 8.

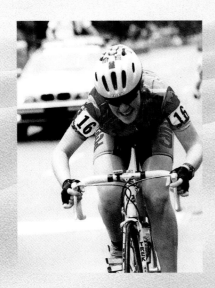

Clara Hughes
C Y C L I N G

Born in Winnipeg, Manitoba, Clara now lives in Hamilton, Ontario, and has been a member of the Canadian national team since 1991. She had a big year in 1995, taking two 1sts in the Tour de l'Aude in France, 1sts in the Canadian championships and the World Cup and 2nds in the world championships and the Pan American Games. Clara is a full-time athlete with the Saturn racing team. She enjoys reading in her spare time.

Nutritional values per serving
(based on 8 servings):
calories: 265
fat: 4 g; 15% of calories
protein: 7 g; 11% of calories
carbohydrates: 49 g; 74% of calories

Clara's Performance Eating Tip:

The key to good health is balance and moderation. It's okay to eat treats—just not every day.

Kelli's Chocolate Cheesecake

Preparation time: 3 hours

Kelli loves chocolate and coffee — one bite of this, and she's on a sugar high for hours.

Crust:

1 Tbsp.	sugar	15 mL
1¼ cups	graham cracker crumbs	300 mL
¼ cup	melted butter	50 mL

Butter sides and bottom of 10-inch (3 L) springform pan. Combine sugar and crumbs. Shake enough crumbs into pan to coat bottom and sides. Add melted butter to remaining crumbs, blend, and press into pan.

Filling:

1 lb.	softened cream cheese	500 g
1 cup	sugar	250 mL
4	eggs	4
2 tsp.	vanilla	10 mL
½ cup	hot brewed coffee	125 mL
12 oz.	semisweet chocolate	375 g

Preheat oven to 325°F (160°C). Beat cream cheese until fluffy and light. Add sugar, and beat, then beat in eggs one at a time. Stir in vanilla. In a separate bowl, mix together hot coffee and chocolate until chocolate is melted, then combine with cream-cheese mixture. Pour into pan, and bake for 55 minutes. Turn off heat, and let stand in oven for 2-3 hours. Serve topped with whipped cream and chipped chocolate. Serves 12.

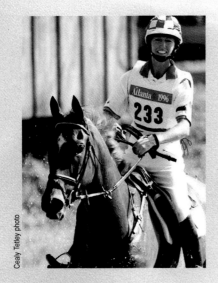

Cealy Tetley photo

Kelli McMullen-Temple
E Q U E S T R I A N

Kelli began riding with the Charlotte Pony Club in Vermont. In 1989, her horse Macavity won the U.S. Combined Training Association's Horse of the Year award. In 1994, Kelli was the USCTA's leading female rider, and her horse King's Revenge won Horse of the Year. The same year, she was 3rd overall in the Land Rover FEI North American three-day-event rider rankings. In 1995, she was 2nd in the USCTA Rider of the Year standings.

Kelli, who has dual Canadian-U.S. citizenship, began riding for Canada in 1995. She was the only Canadian rider to qualify two horses for the 1996 Olympics.

Kelli's Performance Eating Tip:

If you love sweets, don't deny yourself—just remember that moderation is the key.

Nutritional values per serving
(based on 12 servings; without whipped cream or chipped chocolate):
calories: 462
fat: 30 g; 58% of calories
protein: 7 g; 6% of calories
carbohydrates: 42 g; 36% of calories

Chocolate Sorbet

Preparation time: 45 minutes

Eric loves this dessert because it is a treat for the taste buds and a great way to cool down after an intense workout.

1 cup	sugar	250 mL
3¼ cups	water	800 mL
½ cup	light corn syrup	125 mL
3 oz.	semisweet chocolate	75 g
1½ cups	cocoa powder	375 mL
4 tsp.	rum (optional)	20 mL

Boil sugar, corn syrup and 1¼ cups (300 mL) water in saucepan until sugar is dissolved. Remove from heat, and cool. Melt chocolate in double boiler. Place all ingredients except 2 cups (500 mL) water in a large bowl, and whisk together until smooth. Whisk remaining water into mixture, and strain to remove any lumps. Place in ice-cream maker until set, and store in freezer until needed. Serves 6 generously.

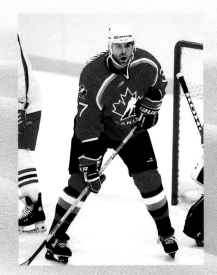

Eric Desjardins
H O C K E Y

Eric is a 28-year-old native of Rouyn, Quebec, and is a key player for the Philadelphia Flyers, whom he joined after 6½ seasons with the Montreal Canadiens. A 1993 Stanley Cup champion, he has also played on the NHL All-Stars (1992, 1996) and the NHL Second All-Stars (1994, 1995). In 1995, he was awarded the Barry Ashbee Trophy.

Nutritional values per serving
(based on 6 servings):
calories: 386
fat: 8 g; 18% of calories
protein: 5 g; 5% of calories
carbohydrates: 73 g; 75 % of calories

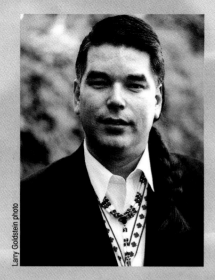

David Wolfman
A B O R I G I N A L
C U L I N A R Y T E A M

David cooked his first meal for his mother when he was ten. Since then, he has honed his craft and learned about Aboriginal culture. He has been the chef for many fine kitchens, including the National Club, and Marriot hotels.

In 1992, he was Captain of the Aboriginal Culinary Team sent to the Culinary Olympics in Frankfurt. The team returned with an impressive seven gold medals, two silver, and two bronze. In May of 1997, he was invited to be the executive chef for the Sacred Assembly Celebration Dinner in Ottawa. He is a professor of Aboriginal Cuisine at George Brown College in Toronto.

Nutritional values per serving (based on 6 servings):
calories: 178
fat: 3 g; 15% of calories
protein: 3 g; 8% of calories
carbohydrates: 34 g; 78 % of calories

Blackberry Cobbler

Preparation time: 30 minutes

This dish is reminiscent of David's heritage. He has fond memories of his mother picking berries and using them to prepare tasty dishes such as this one.

⅓ cup	sugar	75 mL
1 tsp.	cornstarch	5 mL
1	medium nectarine, cut into ½-inch pieces	1
1 cup	blackberries	250 mL
1 cup	all-purpose flour	250 mL
1 tsp.	baking powder	5 mL
½ tsp.	salt	2 mL
2½ tsp.	margarine	12 mL
¼ cup	2% milk	50 mL
2 tsp.	slivered almonds	10 mL

Preheat oven to 375°F (190°C). Whisk sugar and cornstarch together in a bowl, mix in fruit, and let rest. In another bowl, combine flour, baking powder and salt, and blend well. Add margarine, and blend until smooth. Gradually stir in milk until the mixture reaches a doughy texture. Place fruit mixture in a 9-inch (23 cm) greased pan. Make 6 oval dumplings, place on top of fruit, and sprinkle with slivered almonds. Bake for 20 minutes. Serve hot. Serves 6.

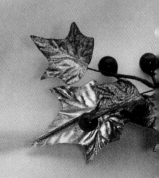

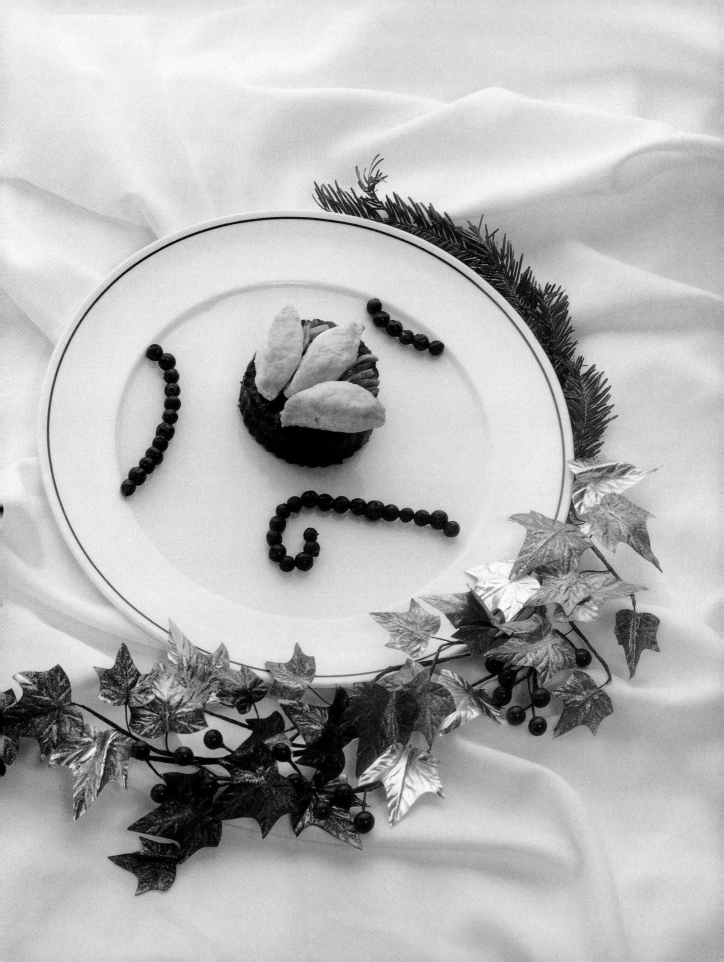

Index of Athletes

Index of Recipes